Life Is Your
BEST MEDICINE

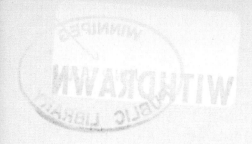

Life Is Your
BEST MEDICINE

A Woman's Guide to
Health, Healing, and Wholeness
at Every Age

Tieraona Low Dog, M.D.

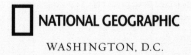

NATIONAL GEOGRAPHIC
WASHINGTON, D.C.

Published by the National Geographic Society
1145 17th Street N.W., Washington, D.C. 20036

ISBN: 978-1-4262-1455-4 (paperback)
First paperback printing 2014

The Library of Congress has cataloged the hardcover edition as follows:

Low Dog, Tieraona.
 Life is your best medicine : a woman's guide to health, healing, and wholeness at every age / Tieraona Low Dog ; foreword by Andrew Weil.
    p. cm.
 ISBN 978-1-4262-0960-4 (hardcover : alk. paper)
 1. Women--Health and hygiene--Popular works. 2. Diet--Popular works. 3. Exercise--Popular works. 4. Self-care, Health--United States--Popular works. I. Title.
 RA778.L68 2012
 613'.04244--dc23
                    2012011775

Cover: National Geographic Photographer Rebecca Hale. Mediterranean Diet Pyramid, p. 50: (cookies) Nikola Bilic/Shutterstock; (beef) Stuart Monk/Shutterstock; (chicken) Senol Yaman/Shutterstock; (eggs) Valentyn Volkov/Shutterstock; (cheese) Nattika/Shutterstock; (yogurt) Africa Studio/Shutterstock; (fish) Andy Lidstone/Shutterstock; (shrimp) Richard Griffin/Shutterstock; (vegetables, nuts, legumes) Mandy Godbehear/Shutterstock; (spice in jar) Madlen/Shutterstock; (olive oil) Valentyn Volkov/Shutterstock; (man running) Flashon Studio/Shutterstock; (man biking) Olly/Shutterstock; (woman practicing yoga) Yuri Arcurs/Shutterstock; (wine) drKaczmar/Shutterstock; (water) artjazz/Shutterstock.

The National Geographic Society is one of the world's largest nonprofit scientific and educational organizations. Founded in 1888 to "increase and diffuse geographic knowledge," the Society's mission is to inspire people to care about the planet. It reaches more than 400 million people worldwide each month through its official journal, *National Geographic,* and other magazines; National Geographic Channel; television documentaries; music; radio; films; books; DVDs; maps; exhibitions; live events; school publishing programs; interactive media; and merchandise. National Geographic has funded more than 10,000 scientific research, conservation and exploration projects and supports an education program promoting geographic literacy.

For more information, visit www.nationalgeographic.com.

National Geographic Society
1145 17th Street N.W.
Washington, D.C. 20036-4688 U.S.A.

For information about special discounts for bulk purchases, please contact
National Geographic Books Special Sales: ngspecsales@ngs.org

For rights or permissions inquiries, please contact National Geographic
Books Subsidiary Rights: ngbookrights@ngs.org

Interior design: Melissa Farris

Printed in the United States of America
14/WOR/1

*To the women who gave me the courage to follow my own
medicine path:
my grandmothers, Josephine and Jessie;
my mother, Vivian;
my teacher, Juba;
and my beautiful daughter, Kiara.
Your strength and love flow through me, inspiring all
that I do. I am forever in your debt.*

Contents

Foreword

The first time I heard Dr. Tieraona Low Dog lecture I knew she was special—a charismatic and caring physician with an unusual breadth and depth of knowledge. It was 1996, when we were both on the faculty of a course on botanical medicine for health professionals offered at Columbia University. I had studied botany before I went to medical school, and this has long been a field of particular interest to me. For many years, I recommended herbal remedies to patients with good results, but I had met very few doctors proficient in the use of herbs and other natural treatments. Listening to Dr. Low Dog was exciting. I marveled at her boundless energy and enthusiasm and was in awe of her ability to cite innumerable research studies from memory. I thought to myself, "I would love to work with her."

Years later my wish came true when Tieraona joined the faculty of the Arizona Center for Integrative Medicine. She assumed the key role of Director of the Fellowship—our intensive training program for doctors, nurse practitioners, and medical residents. She soon became an outstanding leader and beloved teacher. We now frequently share the podium to teach about medicinal plants, culinary herbs and spices, dietary influences on health, and other topics that we both enjoy. We also work together to design and formulate innovative natural products to promote good health.

Because we've spent a lot of quality time in each other's company, I thought I knew Tieraona Low Dog—until I read this book. *Life Is Your Best Medicine* is not only a comprehensive and highly practical guide for women seeking optimum health, it is also Tieraona's own life story, sparkling with the wisdom she has drawn from it. I had no idea of all the adventures she had and the diverse experiences that made her the person she is today. The title of the book conveys the essence of her teaching: Your own experience is an invaluable and trustworthy source of information about how to maintain health as you go through life and deal with the common problems you encounter.

Until very recently, the medical profession excluded women, and even when medical schools began admitting them, the profession remained a male-dominated guild for a long time. Male physicians, often paternalistic and authoritarian, told female patients what to do, and women did not question their prescriptions. For most of the 20th century, they rejected herbs and natural therapies not covered in conventional medical education, dismissed many female complaints as hysterical or psychosomatic, and promoted dangerous treatments, such as hysterectomy for minor uterine problems and hormone replacement therapy for every menopausal patient. They most certainly did not encourage women to take charge of their bodies and health and be guided by their life experience.

Ironically, women are much more health conscious than men in our society. They take better care of themselves and are more likely to seek professional help for symptoms that demand attention. Women are the chief buyers of books about health and self-care, and women's magazines have been major outlets for information on these subjects. Over the past few decades, women have led the consumer movement for holistic and alternative medicine, because they are more open than men to natural therapies, mind/body interventions, and the healing traditions of other cultures. That consumer movement, which is still gaining strength, laid the foundation for acceptance of integrative medicine.

Women's health risks and concerns are different from those of men. The female reproductive system is more complex than its male counterpart; more can go wrong with it, and the array of hormones that regulate its function strongly affect other organs, including the brain. Women are much more likely to develop autoimmune diseases and depression. As the caregivers in our society, they are subject to greater and different forms of stress. Because women have been mostly excluded as test subjects in research studies, gender differences in responses to drugs are significant, and in many cases, unknown.

For all of these reasons, women need special guidance about maintaining health as they journey through life. They need to know about effects of lifestyle choices, the influence of diet on disease risks, the importance of regular physical activity, and ways to protect their bodies and minds from the harmful effects of stress. They also need to know when and how to use preventive medical services, when to seek help from conventional doctors, and when alternative treatments and natural remedies may be appropriate.

This book answers those needs. Dr. Low Dog is a trustworthy source of information that she has gathered from her academic studies as well as her life experience. I can think of no one better qualified to guide women to health, healing, and wholeness at any age.

Andrew Weil, M.D.
Tucson, Arizona
April 2012

Preface

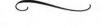

Two roads diverged in a yellow wood . . .
I took the one less traveled by,
And that has made all the difference.
—ROBERT FROST

The word *medicine* is derived from the Latin *medicina,* which means to heal, or to restore to health. In modern times, the word *medicine* is almost always associated with prescription drugs and to a lesser extent with doctors, nurses, and surgery. Although these are important, medicine, when viewed in this way, becomes reactionary, seeing and treating everything as a disease. If medicine is really about healing and health, we must begin to view it in a much broader light. Human beings are complex creatures living in a complex environment. There is no magic pill or supplement for much of what ails us. True healing can only be found in the way we live our lives, which includes our relationships, thoughts, and beliefs.

I am not alone in this perspective. The evidence is overwhelmingly clear that most of the chronic disease we are confronting in the United States has its roots in the way we live our lives. Despite the widespread availability of pharmaceutical medications, advanced surgical care, and state-of-the-art medical technology, more than 50 percent of the

American population is chronically ill. Although life expectancy has increased dramatically over the past hundred years, it's shocking that experts predict future generations of our children are unlikely to live as long as their grandparents. And many of us who live into our elder years will be confronted with debilitating age-related illness that will reduce the quality of our life.

Research shows that if Americans embraced a healthier way of living—a balance between rest and exercise, wholesome nutrition, healthy weight, positive social interactions, stress management, no smoking, limited alcohol use, and limited or no exposure to toxic chemicals—93 percent of diabetes, 81 percent of heart attacks, 50 percent of strokes, and 36 percent of all cancers could be prevented! Unfortunately, most health care providers don't receive any training in how to motivate and help people make the changes necessary to reduce their risk for disease. And let's be clear: Based on the best of the scientific evidence, there isn't any drug on the market that can come close to the power of a healthy lifestyle in preventing disease and improving the quality of our lives. The power to experience vitality and well-being lies within each of us.

Another area that deeply concerns me is the growing numbers of individuals being placed on medications for attention deficit/hyperactivity disorder (ADHD), depression, and anxiety. In 2010, one in ten Americans over the age of 12 were on antidepressants and more than 40 million of us were taking antianxiety drugs. We're told our sadness and tension are due to abnormal levels of brain chemicals and that drugs can return them to their optimal state. Yet, exhaustive reviews of the scientific data published in the *Journal of the American*

Medical Association and the *New England Journal of Medicine* show that these medications are no more effective than a sugar pill for all but the most severe forms of depression.

The growing influence of pharmaceutical companies and direct-to-consumer advertising—along with the lack of training of health care providers in nondrug treatments for depression and anxiety and the inability of people to deal with the overwhelming stress in their lives—has led us to become a nation that turns to pills for our happiness. Yet, as you will see throughout this book, there is strong evidence we can improve our emotional health through exercise, nutrition, good social relationships, positive coping skills, adequate sleep, and relaxation strategies.

The biggest health challenge facing us today is trying to figure out how to live a balanced life. I don't mean a life without ups and downs but rather one that is resilient during change. Resilient people are able to gather their strength and resources to overcome adversity. We're most able to do this when we are physically, emotionally, and spiritually nourished. When women tell me they're too busy to exercise, cook, or make time for themselves, I use it as an opportunity to explore what's really important to them. Because if you think you're too busy to do those things that will lessen your risk of chronic disease and premature death, I'd say it's probably time to reevaluate and reprioritize your life.

I'm grateful for all the opportunities I've been given to taste the fruits of many healing traditions over the years: massage therapy, midwifery, herbalism, and Western, or conventional, medicine. I believe they have made me a better physician, teacher, mother, and friend. My mind and body were enriched from years of practicing tae kwon do, a Korean martial art. I have found wisdom in the teachings of Jesus and within Buddhist philosophy and have sought to make peace with my shadow self through meditation, vision quests, and ritual. I strive to live without regret and be gentle with my imperfect and evolving soul. I've learned during the first half century of my life that my health is deeply affected by my thoughts and beliefs. When I believe that I'm strong and capable and worthy of love, that's what I bring into my world.

This book is a collection of my thoughts and ideas evolved over the span of my life; they have deeply influenced my work as a physician. At first glance, some of the essays might seem puzzling in a book about medicine and health, but I believe that as your reading unfolds, you will begin to see that indeed the everyday stuff of our lives influences our ability to be healthy and whole. In the long run, *life is your best medicine.*

Part I

THE MEDICINE

OF

MY LIFE

The cave you fear to enter holds the treasures you seek.

—JOSEPH CAMPBELL

WHEN I WAS A GIRL, my Grandma Jo told me that when we're born, we're set upon a path and that path is our medicine road. Our entire life, she said, is about learning to be human. All the choices we make along the way affect our thoughts, our relationships, our health, and the world around us. I guess this way of viewing life resonated with me at a young age, as I've never thought of life any other way. I believe everything that happens serves some purpose, even though we can usually only understand it when we're looking back—it's hard to see how it will all come together looking forward. It's not easy learning to be a human being.

I was born in Oklahoma to good parents, baptized in a Methodist church, and for those of you interested in such things, I'm a Sagittarius. I come from midwestern roots, and like most Americans, I'm of mixed heritage: Irish, English, Comanche, Lakota, and a smattering of French and German somewhere in the family tree. I was extremely close to both of my grandmothers, Jo and Jessie, and my paternal grandfather, Glenn. My maternal grandfather was a man of violent temper who never wanted anything to do with me, and although that was painful when I was young, ultimately the feeling was mutual. My early years were both happy and challenging. I had difficulties speaking and reading, so my parents took me to the local United Way to get advice. I was diagnosed with a mild speech impediment and dyslexia, a learning disorder that makes it hard to comprehend written language.

It didn't take long for me to start speaking correctly, but dyslexia is a lifelong problem, and I found school stressful. I was smart and able to catch on to concepts quickly, but reading and writing didn't come easily. I managed pretty well in elementary school by learning to pay close attention to the pictures and illustrations in books that would give me clues about the story or topic. I developed strong listening skills and was blessed with a good memory. I remembered the words people said in the form of snapshots. Not only could I repeat almost verbatim what my teacher said, but I could also tell you where she was standing and what she was wearing when she said it. Still, school was an anxiety-provoking place. My fourth-grade homeroom teacher liked taking kids out in the hall and paddling them if he didn't think they were working hard enough in class. I felt terrified when he'd call on me to read or spell out loud. He shamed and embarrassed me when I'd mix up words and letters.

Like many kids with dyslexia, I excelled in classes that involved discussion and critical thinking. One of my favorite teachers in junior high school used the lyrics of popular songs, particularly those of Simon and Garfunkel, to teach English. But junior high also brought endless amounts of reading, essay writing, and advanced math. My algebra teacher, the football coach, didn't teach; he just assigned problems. I was lost as I tried to make sense of the letters and numbers that had been my adversaries for most of my life. I was working harder and falling further behind.

I started ditching the hard classes, living in fear of what would happen when my parents found out. I experimented with drugs, medicating away my feelings of failure. My parents were at a loss how to help, telling me I was smart and just needed to work harder, which, though they didn't intend it, made me feel even more stupid and lazy. Finally, they sold my beautiful horse and friend Bo, a gift from my Grandma Jo, for what they believed were all the right reasons: I was having trouble caring for him as school took up more and more time, and by ditching classes, I wasn't demonstrating responsibility. But losing Bo broke my heart and left me devastated. My self-esteem and confidence withered—it was as if I were walking barefoot on glass. I dropped out of school when I was 16, and left home with no clear path of where I was going or what I was going to do.

I wandered for the next two years, moving in with a guy I'd known in high school and working at a meatpacking plant outside Amarillo, Texas. But I grew restless and moved on, picking up minimum-wage jobs at places like Pizza Inn and McDonald's as I hung out at powwows and multitribal gatherings in Oklahoma and South Dakota. I made friends and listened to what others were willing to share about their lives, all the while trying to find what was missing in mine.

I was drawn to the culture and ceremonies of the Plains tribes, particularly the Comanche and Lakota, having been exposed to them in my youth. Praying with other women in the sweat lodge connected me to a deeply feminine part of myself. An elder Lakota man, Thomas, who shared my love of horses, told me stories about his life as a boy, and about gentling horses and healing herbs. American Indian activism was on the rise in the 1970s, as outspoken leaders brought attention to the many injustices that continued to be perpetuated on their people. My eyes were opened in many important ways. After a time, though, I realized that whatever I was looking for, it wasn't to be found in the towns and reservations of Oklahoma and the northern plains. Although I shared a common ancestry with some of the Native American people there, it wasn't my home.

I traveled to Richmond, Virginia, where my parents had moved for work. I stayed with them for a time, but we'd been apart too long to feel comfortable living in the same house again. I got a job doing temporary office work and moved out. I dabbled in leatherwork, apprenticing with an old saddle-maker, Frank, and I saved enough money to open my own shop, engraving custom-made saddles and making leather goods. That's where I met Juba, a midwife and Jamaican by birth who had come in looking for someone to make her a beaded leather medicine bag.

Within Juba's large, 40ish-year-old frame lived the biggest heart of anyone I'd ever met. I felt instantly safe with and connected to her. I told her my great-grandmother had helped deliver babies and that I knew a bit about herbal medicine, and then I asked if I could go with her to a birth someday. She laughed and told me that midwifery was illegal in Virginia, but if I wanted to come along she'd be happy for the help. No one bothered Juba because she only caught babies in the

Church Hill district of Richmond, one of the ten most dangerous neighborhoods in the country.

Juba generously shared her knowledge of the ancient woman arts with me, teaching me about herbs, pregnancy, and birth. I was thirsty and drank deeply from the well of her knowing. She supported my taking massage classes as she thought that healers and midwives should know the art of kneading and rubbing.

Life was going along pretty well, but I was struggling financially. My leather shop barely paid the bills. Training with Juba didn't bring in money, and I had to pay for massage classes. I moved into a little room on Grace Street, where I shared a bathroom and kitchen with others living on the same floor. Every day on my way to catch the bus to Church Hill and Juba, I walked by the Kim School of Tae Kwon Do. Little did I know then that, within those walls, my life would be changed forever.

In exchange for two gymnastic mats that I made, I started taking classes three times each week. I wasn't particularly athletic or flexible, and the training was very demanding. I thought often of quitting. But gradually, over several months, I fell in love with my classes and started helping out around the school. Eventually, I was paid to run the front office. I closed my leather shop and slowly stopped working with Juba, as my passion for tae kwon do consumed me. I was taking an average of 13 to 15 90-minute classes every week and watched in wonder as I pushed my body to the very edge of its limits. My mind became disciplined and focused. I learned to meditate and do yoga. For the first time in my life, I felt like I was really good at something.

I was thriving. I dived deeper into herbal medicine, taking classes from local herbalists, reading any book I could find, and making ointments and teas for my classmates and their families. And it was at the school that I fell deeply in love with Daniel. He was Master Kim's lead black belt and a highly gifted martial artist and teacher. In 1980, we married.

Life was good. For about two years, Daniel and I ran the school together. I'd earned my first-degree black belt by then and loved teaching classes. Then in early 1982, we packed up our two dogs and moved to Sacramento, California, to train with Master Kim's teacher, Grand Master Myung Kyu Kang, one of only three living people in the world to hold the rank of tenth-degree black belt in Moo Duk Kwan Tae Kwon Do, a rank few people ever achieve because of the many decades of training required. He was a wise, gentle, and powerful man who made us feel welcome.

When he learned, shortly after we arrived, that I was pregnant, he invited me to study tai chi with him. I missed the raw power and speed of tae kwon do, but the gentle, flowing movements of tai chi seemed perfect nourishment for the child growing within me. My son, Mekoce, which means "country" or "land" in Lakota, was born in August 1982.

When he was six weeks old, we moved to Las Cruces, New Mexico, so Daniel could teach martial arts at New Mexico State University. We opened a tae kwon do school shortly after our arrival, and I earned my second-degree black belt, taught tae kwon do and tai chi classes three nights a week, and ran a small health food store during the day. Mekoce was the center of my life. He'd been born a beautiful, tender soul. He spent his days at work with me, and Daniel would watch him the nights I was teaching. We were a happy family, living a happy life . . .

Until the moment I learned Daniel had been unfaithful. I was standing behind the counter in our tae kwon do school when I found out. It was as if all the oxygen had been sucked out of the air. I couldn't breathe. When the reality of it finally sank in, I picked up Mekoce, packed our clothes and a few possessions, and left. I never went back.

The divorce played on all my old insecurities. I felt unattractive, unwanted, and embarrassed that my marriage had failed. I didn't know how to grieve the death of my family or mend the betrayal I felt so deep inside. And there was no time to figure it out because, like many single mothers, I had to find a way to support my little boy and me. A chiropractor rented me space in her office, and I started an herbal consulting practice and occasionally taught herb classes at the local food cooperative. Still, I was just getting by financially. I felt sad and overwhelmed by my circumstances. I was lost again, my confidence shaken. It was 1985, and the year I began to prepare for my vision quest.

Will Windbird was one of the people who would come see me now and then for herbal remedies. About 50 years old, he was a tall, lean, gentle man of mixed native and white heritage. He worked at the local prison as a counselor for incarcerated Native American men, and he invited me to talk to his group there about herbs and healing. Will and I became friends, and I appreciated his counsel. So when he suggested that I do a vision quest to find out where my life was taking me, I agreed, thinking it might help me heal the empty place in my heart. I spent the year fasting one day a week, drinking herbal teas to cleanse my body, and praying in the sweat lodge to prepare myself for going out alone for three days and two nights without food or water. The preparation gave me a focus, something to hold on to.

About two months before my vision quest, I dreamed I was riding a big black horse when I came upon a raging river. I carefully tucked all my possessions into a sack and strapped it to my chest so it wouldn't be lost as we crossed. The horse was a powerful swimmer, but the currents were strong and ripped me from his back. The rapids threw me downstream. I couldn't keep my head above water, and my lungs were on fire. I was drowning. Just when I thought I was going to die, the river let me up for air, and above me was a red-tailed hawk on a tree branch hanging low over the water. I heard him say, "To live, you must let go of the sack." I woke in a panic. It was one of those dreams where it takes a minute to realize that it was just that, a dream.

When I shared the story with Will, he thought about it for a bit and then said that I should give away the thing I valued most before going out alone to the desert. Mekoce and I didn't have much, so it didn't seem like that would be hard to do. I knew in my heart that the only thing I didn't want to give away was the piece of jewelry around my neck. The necklace that Thomas, the old man in South Dakota, gave me the last time I'd seen him before he died. Long before I'd met Daniel, Thomas told me I'd give birth to a strong and gentle son, and he told me to name him Mekoce. He told me the necklace would give me strength in the darkness. It was my only connection to him and that part of my life. I wept when I gave it away.

The need to begin the vision quest was getting stronger. I'd gone out to an old ranch and hiked around until I found my "place" in a small exposed area of desert near a wash, with a wall of granite enclosing the north and west sides of a narrow canyon. I went back once again before my quest and spent the day in meditation. It felt right. It was early May when I drove there at dawn and hiked into the canyon. I used the heel of my boot to make a circle about 12 feet across, where I'd spend the next three days. Then I smudged the circle and myself with sage and cedar, the aroma reminding me of the seriousness of what I was about to do. I took off my boots, sat in the center of the circle, and offered tobacco to the spirits of the land.

I spent the next two nights and three mornings in solitude. The sun was merciless. The first night was cold, and I was afraid of the darkness and of animals, snakes, and the demons that haunted my dreams. I didn't sleep. The second day was hot and I was thirsty, but I had no water. Doubts were setting in. How was doing this going to change anything? I thought about leaving or moving my circle to the shade. Isn't that who I was anyway, a quitter? I'd quit high school, I'd quit the friendships of my youth, I'd quit apprenticing with the saddle maker, my leather shop had been a failure, and I'd quit training with Juba. I had no money, my family was far away, and I was trying to raise a little boy all by myself. I hadn't wanted the divorce, didn't expect it, and yet there it was. Out there in the heat of the sun, with nowhere to hide, I felt so exposed and broken.

I thought I had come here in search of my life, but as night fell for the second time, I realized that I was really seeking my death and that giving away the necklace was about letting go of my attachment and need to hold on to stuff. But it wasn't just physical things that I had to let go of. What I symbolically carried in the sack I had strapped close and tight to my chest in my dream was the part of me that carried the shame, the pity, the blame, the pain, and the sorrow of my life. I had to let that part of me die before the woman waiting inside could be born. At some point during the night I fell asleep, exhausted.

And then I felt a presence behind me. To this day I don't know if I was awake or dreaming, but I was so frightened. With my mind, not my ears, I heard the words "I have been with you always." I thought it was God. I started crying, because it seemed like such a long time since I'd felt his presence in my life. I said out loud, "But I couldn't find you." Then softly and gently I heard, "I have been with you always. You just need to turn around."

With the sun barely creeping over the horizon, I laid in my circle looking up at the sky. I believed I could feel my heartbeat in the earth below me. I saw a deer near the mouth of the canyon. She looked over at me and then put her head down and continued to eat. I closed my eyes and said the 23rd Psalm. I felt such peace. I was ready to turn around. I was ready to let go. I was willing to die so that I could be reborn. A song I'd never heard came to my lips, and I knew that it was my medicine song.

My life has had many twists and turns since then, and there have been good times and bad. But I left that circle strong and I left it whole. I studied and earned my GED, and all kinds of doors opened before me.

An older woman I'd helped with herbs co-signed a $15,000 loan so that I could start Tieraona's Herbals, a small herbal manufacturing company. Because I was using local herbs, the New Mexico Department of Agriculture paid for me to showcase my products at two large trade shows in California and England. I moved out of the chiropractor's clinic and opened my own office, where I treated about 30 people a week, using herbs, diet, and massage. I taught tae kwon do for a couple of semesters at the university and started running an herb school out of my office.

Mekoce remained the center of my world. He was a smart and curious child. He loved to watch videos of Care Bears and He-Man and sing along as I played guitar. We were vegetarians, and he liked helping me cook dinner. On the weekends, we'd go hiking or camping in the Organ Mountains outside Las Cruces. I remember moving the furniture out of the living room and teaching an eight-week tai chi class at our house to make enough extra money to buy him a pair of Air Jordan tennis shoes for Christmas. He loved those shoes so much that I had to pry them off his feet at bedtime. We were happy and things were going well. But once again, the direction of my life was about to change.

One evening as I was closing up my office, a man came in with a sick baby. It didn't take but a minute to know she was really ill. She cried when I moved her neck, and I thought she might have meningitis. I told the father he had to take her to the hospital. He hesitated and then asked if there were herbs that could lower her fever. I knew he wasn't legally in the country. It was early August, and he was probably one of the workers who'd come to harvest the green chili.

It was after 6 p.m., and I had to pick up Mekoce from after-school care. Feeling pressed for time, I pulled ten dollars out of the cashbox and wrote on a sheet of paper the address for La Clinica De Familia and the word *acetaminophen*. I told him to go to the clinic, where the doctor could help his baby, and reassured him that no one would ask for any kind of papers. I told him to use the money to buy medicine for her fever. I picked up Mekoce, who'd been impatiently waiting, while the teacher glared and reminded me I was late.

A couple of days later, the man came back to my office holding a small bouquet of field flowers. I was happy to see him and smiled as I accepted his gift. In broken English, he told me that he was going back to Mexico with his wife and their baby, who had died in the night. He wanted to thank me for my kindness. I saw a woman in the front seat of an old Ford holding a small bundle in her arms. They drove away.

I could hardly work. I didn't know what to think or what to do. I was angry that he hadn't taken the baby to the doctor and ashamed that I'd been in such a hurry to leave. I felt the enormous weight of not knowing enough and realized the incredible gift and power that a deeper knowledge of medicine could provide. I decided that I wanted to become a doctor.

I studied for and took the ACT exam and then enrolled for classes at New Mexico State. When I went in to see the premed advisor, she encouraged me to get a nursing degree. When I told her I wanted to be a physician, not a nurse, she told me in no uncertain terms that, based on my ACT scores, she didn't think I'd make it.

But the part of me that in the past would have thought, "I'm stupid. She's probably right. I won't be able to do it," had been left behind in that circle in the desert. The woman who'd been born that third morning was strong. She was an herbalist, midwife, massage therapist, teacher, businesswoman, second-degree black belt, tai chi instructor, and mother, and she could do anything she set her mind to. I raised my son and ran my clinic, school, and herbal company while taking 18 credits every semester and maintaining a 3.8 GPA. I was accepted at the University of New Mexico School of Medicine, where I graduated Outstanding Senior Medical Student in 1996.

Over the years, I came to learn that most of the things I once considered failures were really blessings in disguise. If I hadn't dropped out of high school, I never would have met Thomas or felt the magic of the sweat lodge. But if I'd felt at home in the plains, I wouldn't have traveled to Richmond and met Frank, opened my leather shop, and found Juba. She taught me about being a woman, about birth, and mid-wifed me through a critical period of my life. If my leather shop had been successful, I never would have moved down to Grace Street and found the Kim School of Tae Kwon Do. I never would have learned martial arts or studied tai chi with Master Kang. And if I had never met Daniel, my beautiful son wouldn't be in the world and in my life. If the divorce hadn't happened, I'd never have gone on the vision quest, which taught me to let go of the past and embrace my faith again. The strength I found in the desert those three days allowed me to pursue my business, school, and clinical practice, which provided enough money for Mekoce and me to live comfortably. If the migrant worker hadn't come to my clinic and returned to tell me his little girl had died, I never would have thought of becoming a physician. All these links in the chain of my life gave me the tenacity to work my way through college and medical school.

After leaving my residency in family medicine, I opened an integrative medical practice in Albuquerque, where I was able to offer a wide variety of treatment options for my patients. So much of the chronic disease in our country could be prevented through stress management, healthy relationships, a wholesome diet, physical activity, and avoiding exposure to harmful environmental toxins. Unfortunately, there's virtually no training in any of these subjects in medical school. But because of my background, I was able to counsel my patients about medications and surgery and also about nutrition, herbs, exercise, massage, forgiveness, and contentment. I honestly believe that it is in the everyday stuff of our lives that we find the answers to experiencing an emotionally and physically rich life. This is the essence of integrative medicine.

In 2000, President Bill Clinton appointed me to serve on the White House Commission on Complementary and Alternative Medicine Policy, one of my greatest honors. In 2003, Secretary Tommy Thompson of Health and Human Services appointed me to the advisory board of the National Institutes of Health National Center for Complementary and Alternative Medicine, where I served until my appointment ended in 2007. I was nominated and served as chair of the United States Pharmacopeia Dietary Supplements and Botanicals Expert Panel from 2000 to 2010, and now chair its safety subcommittee. I have the privilege of training more than a hundred physicians and nurse practitioners in integrative medicine every year in my role as Fellowship Director at the

Arizona Center for Integrative Medicine, where I also hold the rank of Clinical Associate Professor of Medicine at the University of Arizona Health Sciences Center.

My early difficulties with reading and writing made me highly observant, a skill that has proved useful in identifying wild plants in the field or conducting a thorough physical exam on a patient. And though I'm not a natural writer, I've learned that I don't have to be intimidated by the written word. I've written more than 20 peer-reviewed articles in medical journals, 17 chapters for textbooks, and authored or edited three books. If I didn't have dyslexia, I never would have developed my auditory memory or listening skills. It makes me happy when patients say they felt "heard" when they leave my office. I smile when I think of my early fear of speaking in front of other people. And although I still have difficulty spelling basic words out loud, mixing up *c, k, s, d,* and *t,* it hasn't stopped me from public speaking; I've been an invited lecturer at more than 500 medical and scientific conferences.

I have had many personal blessings along the way. I have fallen in and out of relationships, grateful for what each brought into my life. When I finally learned to be content and happy in my own company, and when I wasn't looking for or expecting it, I discovered the person who would become my best friend and husband. He never so much as blinked as he took care of me when I was being treated for cancer and recovering from hip-replacement surgery. We can stay up talking late into the night or sit for hours together on the back porch without saying anything at all. The days pass by gently on our ranch in northern New Mexico, where we live in a log cabin surrounded by dogs, cats, horses, and 185 acres of forest.

I was blessed to have another child in 1994, the daughter I'd dreamed of for many years. Kiara was born at home, and I knew she was the one I'd been waiting for. Because of my own struggles with school, I was far more willing to be creative with my children's education. Mekoce and Kiara attended public school some years and I homeschooled them others. Mekoce graduated top of his class at the University of New Mexico and completed his master's degree in political science at the University of California, Berkeley. He is fluent in Spanish and nearly so in Italian and French. Kiara, an incredibly gifted writer and avid homeschooler, decided that she'd start college at 15. She's a junior at the University of New Mexico at the ripe old age of 17, majoring in anthropology. My heart feels so full; I thank God every day that he chose me to be the caretaker of these two precious souls.

As I look back across the span of my life, I realize that what I once thought were mistakes were really just events and situations preparing me for what lies ahead. I chose the quote by Joseph Campbell to open this section because it captures the truth of my life and maybe yours, too. "The cave you fear to enter holds the treasures you seek." The cave I feared to enter was my own mind, and I was afraid of what I'd find there. Within that circle in the desert, I thought I feared the wild animals and rattlesnakes that inhabited the land; in truth, I was frightened to peer into the abyss, not knowing what I'd find. But Campbell was right. I found my treasures in the darkness and solitude.

I feel called to the work I do and called to share what I've learned with you. I resisted writing this book for many years, not only because I'm not a writer but also because I didn't know how to capture and organize what I wanted to say.

The answers to our well-being cannot be found by simply taking a prescription drug. So much of modern illness can be prevented or mended with wholesome food, movement, meditation, forgiveness, interaction with nature, and social connectedness. And even in the absence of a cure, we can choose to be healed.

We can't measure healing with a blood pressure cuff or by the values on a lab test. True healing is experienced and measured by our level of contentment and joy. And healing is the essence of this book.

It is my prayer that it may provide some help, some assistance as you journey along your own medicine road.

Part II

HONORING THE BODY

Our bodies are our gardens, to the
which our wills are gardeners.
—WILLIAM SHAKESPEARE

WHAT A PERFECT METAPHOR for how we can relate to our body! There are few things in the world more beautiful than gardens. Those of us who tend them know they require considerable work, and that we get out of it what we put in. We also know that it takes a lot less effort in the long run if our gardens are tended regularly and given what they need to thrive—a balance of sunshine and shade, dryness and moisture, and nutrient-rich soil. If any of these vital components are missing, the seeds we plant will have to compete with weeds for sustenance, the plants will not be as healthy, the flowers less brilliant, and the harvest less bountiful. Those are basically the components we need for taking care of our body. And if we tend it every day, we'll find it doesn't require nearly as much work as we get older.

Our bodies need sunshine and shade, both literally and metaphorically. We need sunshine for vitamin D, which is important not only for our bones but also for our cardiovascular, immune, and nervous systems. But too much sun can increase our risk for skin cancer, so moderation is key. Sunshine and shade also represent activity and rest. We need to be physically active, because our bodies were designed for movement. It keeps our minds sharp, bones healthy, and muscles lean and strong, while reducing our risk for depression, heart disease, diabetes, weight gain, and cancer. At the same time, we need rest, sleep, and dreams for renewal.

Also like plants, our bodies won't thrive in depleted soil. Our "soil" does best when nourished with minimally processed fruits and vegetables, grains, seed oils, nuts, and seeds. Organic dairy, meat from animals humanely raised without antibiotics or hormones, and oily cold-water fish low in mercury can round out our food palette, based on individual preference and taste. We need hydration with clean water, teas, and herbal beverages, and if we choose, an occasional glass of wine. There is tremendous agreement that if we live a life based on these principles, we can give our body an edge against many of the chronic diseases that diminish the quality of our lives.

Yet to live a life of these principles also requires that we manage our stress, choose health, and have a loving relationship with our body. When we're feeling really stressed, our body releases hormones like cortisol that signal a fight-or-flight response. When that happens, we crave pastries, doughnuts, or potato chips—anything high in fat and/or sugar that our body can quickly convert to fuel. High cortisol levels make sleeping more difficult, denying our body the rest it needs and making us feel even more stressed, irritable, and hungry. If we exercise, we can use up some of the fuel that we consumed in response to stress, but many of us under stress come home exhausted and enjoy our favorite television shows instead of exercising because we need an escape. We're no longer running from lions and bears—the things chasing us now are text messages, emails, and never ending demands on our time. We have to learn to manage this stress for our bodies to be in balance.

We need to choose to be healthy. This is important. Please note that I didn't say we must choose to be thin. You can be overweight and healthy as well as thin and unhealthy. This is not about focusing on your body size; it's about choosing to see a healthy body as a resource for accomplishing the things you want to do in life. Nourish your body with wholesome foods because they're better for you, your family, and your world. Be active so your body can move in the world without fatigue or pain. Rest so you can awake refreshed and ready to start the day.

But to do all this often requires a shift in the way we view our body. We women are notorious for examining our body under a microscope and invariably finding it wanting. We save our harshest criticism for our physical form: too flat, too round, too big, too small, too tall, too short. There's a reason we hand over more than $450 billion a year to the weight loss and beauty industries. The message these industries proclaim is that we can always be thinner, prettier, or sexier—that we should never be satisfied with what we've got. I've sat with gorgeous women who told me how much they hated their thighs, breasts, or arms. But think about this: What do you lovingly care for that you hate? Nothing. We only care for the things and people we love.

Your body is your most faithful friend, one of your most valuable resources, the sacred vessel that holds your spirit. I can think of few things more worthy of your devotion.

Breath

*A lifetime is not what is between the
moments of birth and death.
A lifetime is one moment between
my two little breaths.*
—CHADE MENG, TAOIST POET

I had never really given much thought to breathing
until I started taking tae kwon do classes in my late
teens. I mean, what was there to think about? I'd
been breathing all my life.
So it came as quite a shock when I realized that I didn't
know the first thing about breathing correctly, nor did I know
what an amazing tool it could be for maintaining a sense of
calm or enduring hours of rigorous martial arts training.
Worse, like many young women, I sucked in my tummy to
look thin, tightening my abdominal muscles and taking shallow breaths, breathing only from the upper part of my lungs.

At the beginning and end of every tae kwon do class, we
were instructed to sit quietly for three to five minutes, with
eyes closed and focusing on our breath. At first, I was kind of
bored and felt a little stupid. I would open one eye and look
around to see if anyone else was peeking. It seemed silly to sit
there and just breathe. But after a while, I started following
along with the rest of the class, and over the course of several

months, I found that these periods of slow, deep breathing had a profoundly relaxing effect upon me. I began practicing outside class. Inhale for five seconds, let my abdomen relax, exhale for five seconds, and let my abdomen gently contract. I would practice standing in line at the grocery store or while cooking dinner or at night when I was ready to sleep.

Later, when I was studying midwifery, I learned that women could breathe through their contractions, that they could, with practice, labor and bring their babies into the world without medication. It was my breath that allowed me to bring my children into the world—my daughter, Kiara, was born at home with a midwife and no medication. I've witnessed the first breath taken by countless infants, and as a physician, I've witnessed the final breath of those passing over. It's humbling to think that only one breath separates life from death.

Humans have always known that breath is sacred. In Sanskrit texts, the breath is *prana,* which roughly translates as life force. It is said that each of us is allotted a set number of breaths for our time on earth. Both the Hebrew word *ruah* and the Greek word *pneuma* are translated as breath or spirit. Breath prayers— where short lines of scripture, often psalms, were contemplated while taking very slow, deep breaths—were common in ancient times. During times of difficulty, I have personally found great comfort in the 23rd Psalm, saying the words "The Lord is my shepherd" as I inhale and "I shall not want" as I exhale. These words are not spoken out loud; I say them in my mind as they follow the rhythm of my breath. Whatever your personal belief about the divine, there's little doubt that humans have long recognized breath is intricately intertwined with spirit.

I believe that breath work, or breathing exercises, are very powerful tools for maintaining health and well-being. Our lives today are so hurried and filled with stress. I see it every day in my office. Patients complain of neck pain, back pain, stomach problems, anxiety, depression, insomnia, and headaches. We move and stand with shoulders slouched and scrunched, neck tight and rigid. We sit hunched over our desks and computers, answering emails, working on reports, or hunched over our steering wheels, racing to the next appointment.

Stress activates the fight-or-flight response, or to be more exact, it activates the sympathetic nervous system. In really dangerous situations, this response can save our life by releasing hormones such as cortisol and adrenaline, which mobilize the blood sugar and fats we need to run away or fight. These hormones also increase our heart rate and blood pressure, dampen down the immune system, and divert energy away from body functions such as digestion, elimination, and reproduction, because they are not absolutely essential to survive danger. When the stress is over, the parasympathetic nervous system kicks in and the body and mind relax. Blood sugar and fats are stored away, blood pressure and heart rate go down, the immune system is freed to do its job, and digestion, elimination, and reproduction return to normal.

But what happens when we're chronically under stress? To begin with, if cortisol levels stay elevated, the risk of heart disease, hypertension, diabetes, infertility, insomnia, constipation, irritable bowel syndrome, upper respiratory infections, and possibly even cancer increase. What can we do to counter that stress response? The answer is right inside us.

We've all heard the adage, "Take a deep breath and count to ten" when we're upset or angry. That piece of advice reflects the ancient awareness that breath can restore calm.

Breathing is influenced by the autonomic nervous system, and research shows that by consciously altering the rhythm of our breath, we can dramatically influence our emotions. That's because when we breathe slowly, parasympathetic activity is increased, and the sympathetic nervous system is turned way down, so there is less adrenaline and cortisol coursing through our body. In fact, studies have shown that when people with mild high blood pressure use a device that teaches them to breathe slowly (less than ten breaths a minute), they can lower their blood pressure without medication. Other research shows that this kind of breathing can help ease anxiety, irritable bowel syndrome, panic attacks, and pain.

You know this intuitively. Imagine for a moment that you're upset or angry or are hurriedly rushing through your day, your work, your life, racing to get to whatever is in front of you. Notice how your body feels; pay attention to your breathing. Compare this to a time when you're feeling content and relaxed. Imagine what you feel like first thing in the morning after a great night's sleep, when there's nothing pressing on the "to-do" list. What is the quality of your breath?

When your breathing is slow and relaxed, tension and anxiety simply fade away. Taking slow, deep breaths is a simple and highly effective way of relieving stress by activating the parasympathetic nervous system, which slows the heart rate, lowers blood pressure, enhances digestion, and causes muscles to relax.

Over the past 20 years, I've taught many patients breathing exercises because I know they're one of the quickest and easiest ways to calm the mind, relax the body, and center the spirit. At the Arizona Center for Integrative Medicine, where I'm the Fellowship Director, all incoming physicians and nurse practitioners are taught how to do the four-seven-eight breath early in their training. At the end of the two-year program, countless numbers of fellows have told me that this one simple technique has changed their own lives as well as the lives of many of their patients. It's hard to believe that it's not taught in public schools, colleges, or medical training programs. It takes only a couple of minutes, is always readily available, doesn't require any equipment, and is absolutely free.

Breathing exercises in general allow the mind to be completely in the here and now. And it's when we're in the present that we experience calmness and peace, because we're not thinking about past mistakes or worrying about what tomorrow might bring. Integrating this simple practice into our daily life is one of the best gifts we can give ourselves.

R℞ PRESCRIPTION FROM DR. LOW DOG
The Four-Seven-Eight Breath

This breathing exercise is amazingly soothing for the nervous system, and you can do it standing or lying down. For now, though, try it seated, back straight but not rigid, legs uncrossed, hands resting softly on the thighs. Make sure you're comfortable and that you have two to three minutes of uninterrupted time:

- Breathe in slowly and quietly through the nose for the count of four, letting your belly expand, while your chest stays soft and relaxed.
- Hold your breath for the count of seven.
- Open your mouth and exhale audibly and completely for the count of eight.
- This is one breath cycle. Repeat three more times for a total of four breaths.

The more you practice the four-seven-eight breath, the more effective it will be at helping you maintain a sense of calm. For the first month, try doing four breaths morning and night—it will help you go to sleep after a long day. Later, you can extend it to eight breaths.

If you feel a little light-headed when you're starting out, don't worry; it'll pass. Also use this breathing exercise whenever you feel yourself getting upset or angry. Take a deep breath and count four-seven-eight. Do it four times before you react to the situation.

Teach your children this exercise, so they'll have a coping strategy as they travel through life.

Food

*Let your food be your medicine
and your medicine be your food.*
—HIPPOCRATES

I f you want to be healthy, one of the most powerful tools at your disposal is your fork. What you choose to put in your mouth has a direct impact on your long-term risk for developing chronic diseases. According to the American Heart Association, the National Cancer Institute, the World Cancer Research Fund, and the World Health Organization, up to 80 percent of heart disease and a third of all cancers could be prevented with a healthy diet and lifestyle. Those are staggering statistics. If I told you I had a pill that could cut your chances of getting cancer by 30 percent and a heart attack by 80 percent without any harmful side effects, would you take it? Of course you would! Although there's no guarantee that a healthy diet will prevent you from ever getting sick, I think most of us want to do what we can to stack the odds in our favor.

Over the past decades, we have lived through the low-fat, calorie-counting, carb-counting, Atkins, South Beach, Zone, raw foods, caveman (Paleolithic), and Eat Right for Your Blood Type approaches to food. Many foods have been vilified: eggs, meat, fish, bread, cheese, milk, and anything with

R℞ PRESCRIPTION FROM DR. LOW DOG
Eat the Mediterranean Way

Admittedly, it *is* more work to prepare a wholesome meal than to pop a frozen dinner in the microwave, but the primary stress in the kitchen generally comes from not having what you need to make the meal you want to cook. The trick is to plan your shopping. I live 30 minutes from a grocery store, so planning is particularly important. And having a ready supply of basic kitchen ingredients on hand makes every meal easier.

Mediterranean Diet Pyramid

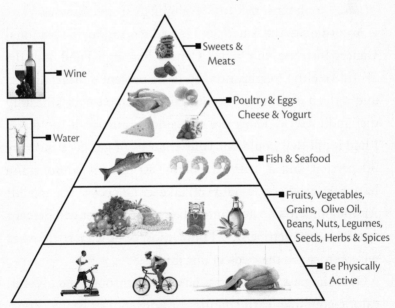

Wine

Water

Sweets & Meats

Poultry & Eggs
Cheese & Yogurt

Fish & Seafood

Fruits, Vegetables, Grains, Olive Oil, Beans, Nuts, Legumes, Seeds, Herbs & Spices

Be Physically Active

The Mediterranean diet is loaded with nutrient-rich vegetables, fruits, whole grains, lean meats, and healthy fats.

sugar. People repeatedly tell me that they're confused by all this. And I tell them that eating healthy isn't that complicated if you understand the basics.

I'm not a certified nutritionist or professional chef. I'm a home cook, mother, and physician. I love delicious food and reject the notion that healthy food equates with boring and bland. In fact, nothing could be further from the truth. My kitchen is stocked with spices, healthy oils, fresh organic fruits and vegetables, whole grains, fish, and humanely raised organic poultry and dairy products. Every time I sit down to eat a meal, I see it as an opportunity to replenish my energy, provide my body with the nutrients it needs to function optimally, and quiet my mind. Food is more than just the sum of its grams of carbohydrates and proteins, calories, vitamins, and minerals. It is a celebration of life, friends, and family.

❦ Family Meals

I like to play soft music, light candles, and set the table nicely for dinner. I treat evening meals as special occasions, because they're our time for family conversation and for catching up on the happenings of the day. This is not the time to argue with our partner or lecture our kids about grades or homework. It's a time to celebrate our togetherness. I'm saddened by the statistics that show many families don't sit down together for even one evening meal a week. Whether the family is two people or a house filled with children, sharing food and conversation is central to healthy relationships.

We're all busy, so adjusting schedules can be a major undertaking, but ensuring that our families eat dinner (or breakfast) together most—or at least some—days of the week can be done if it's important to us. My husband is one of nine children, and his father was a busy vascular surgeon in Omaha, Nebraska. Coordinating dinner for 11 people was no easy task for his mother, given all the after-school activities, the sporting events, and the long working hours of her husband. But both parents made dinnertime a priority.

Children were to be at the table by six—be there or be grounded was the rule! My father-in-law would join the family for dinner before returning to the hospital to do his rounds. This allowed everyone a chance to check in about school and upcoming events and simply to reconnect with one another. Those mealtimes together provided nourishment that went far beyond the content of the food.

Studies repeatedly show that the single strongest factor in higher achievement scores and fewer behavioral problems in children of all ages is having more mealtime at home. A study by Columbia University's National Center on Addiction and Substance Abuse found that teenagers who shared fewer than three dinners a week with their families were almost four times more likely to use tobacco, more than twice as likely to use alcohol, and two and a half times more likely to use marijuana, when compared with teens who had five to seven dinners a week with family. When interviewed, most children report that the interaction and togetherness are the best parts of the meal. The busier our lives become, the more important it is to carve out protected time.

Aside from just eating together, cooking together can be a lot of fun for the whole family. If you don't know how to cook, just get yourself a cookbook, and bring your kids into the kitchen with you. I'm amazed at how many people tell me they don't know how to cook. When I was in junior high school, everyone had to take home economics class. We learned how to cook, create a shopping list, balance the checkbook, as well as perform rudimentary sewing and basic child care. As a girl, I helped my mother and my grandmothers in the kitchen and absolutely loved making homemade cookies, pies, and cakes during my preteen years. I taught my children how to cook when they were young, inviting them to help me make the salad, cook the rice, steam the veggies, and set the table. Children are far less picky about their food when they help prepare it. Teaching kids to cook is a natural way to teach them healthy eating habits, and studies show that teens get about 71 percent of their health information from their mothers and about 43 percent from their fathers.

When my kids were still in school and living at home, we started our meals with a prayer, quote, or poem. We took turns with this from day to day, and when it was our daughter, Kiara's, turn, she would read from *A Grateful Heart: Daily Blessings for the Evening Meal from Buddha to the Beatles,* a fabulous little book that reflected her eclectic teenage spirit. The intention of the reading or prayer was to have a clear demarcation between the busyness of the day and the celebration of our family and our food.

Although we usually ate dinner at the table, there were occasions when we made a homemade whole wheat pizza or sandwiches and watched a movie or TV show together.

When Kiara went through her phase of loving *American Idol,* we would put our food on trays and watch the semifinals together in the living room, each of us voting for our favorite contestant. These were definitely "date nights" that we all looked forward to. OK, well, my husband, Jim, didn't exactly look forward to watching that particular show, but he was a good sport and joined in! Sometimes, when the weather was nice, we would make a picnic and sit outside on the porch. The birds made soft music, and the trees served as a delightful backdrop for the meal.

Now that the children are grown, Jim helps me in the kitchen, chopping onions and vegetables as we catch up on the day, share a glass of wine, and listen to relaxing music. We set the table, light the candles, and have long conversations about all kinds of things as we eat. These dinners fortify our relationship and help keep our marriage strong.

If you are finding family meals difficult to achieve, try starting with Sunday brunch or dinner. After a while, you can pick an additional night that works with everyone's schedule.

❦ Healthy Whole Food

Food is healthiest when it's as close to nature as possible. Processed foods are stripped of key nutrients and then are loaded with preservatives, salt, high-fructose corn syrup (HFCS), sweeteners, trans fats, artificial flavorings, and colorings. So not only are we losing an incredible array of healthy vitamins, minerals, and fiber when we eat these foods, but we're getting lots of added calories and chemicals. Contrary to what many people believe, whole foods are cheaper than processed. A bag of brown rice or a bunch of carrots are cheaper than prepackaged rice mixes or frozen vegetables in sauce.

R̲X̲ PRESCRIPTION FROM DR. LOW DOG
What's in My Kitchen

Here are some of my basic kitchen staples. You can make your own variations, particularly if you're vegetarian, vegan, or have special dietary needs, like gluten- or dairy-free foods.

- Extra-virgin olive oil, organic expeller-pressed canola oil, lightly toasted sesame oil, and possibly grape seed oil
- Balsamic and rice vinegar
- Soy sauce (low-sodium and naturally fermented or brewed)
- Canned organic chopped tomatoes and tomato sauce
- Frozen organic spinach, green beans, broccoli, peas, shelled edamame, and blueberries
- Whole grain pastas
- Brown and basmati rice
- Quinoa, couscous, millet, and rolled oats
- Canned and dried black beans and red kidney beans, and dried lentils
- Organic chicken and/or vegetable broth
- Unbleached, unbromated white flour and whole wheat flour
- Baking powder and soda, aluminum-free
- Walnuts, almonds, and pine nuts

- Dried fruits such as apricots, figs, cranberries, golden raisins
- A variety of seasonings and spices: Italian seasoning, Mexican seasoning, curry and turmeric powder, cumin, thyme, chili powder, pure vanilla extract, black pepper, salt, cinnamon, nutmeg, ginger, cloves
- Prepared mustard
- Onions and garlic bulbs
- Cane sugar, brown sugar, honey, and maple syrup
- Whole grain breakfast cereals
- Plain yogurt, hard cheeses like pecorino or Parmesan
- Organic milk and/or soy or almond milk
- Organic butter
- Eggs, free-range
- Fresh fruits and vegetables (locally grown and/or organic when possible)
- Humanely raised organic meats and poultry
- Seafood such as sardines or wild Alaska salmon
- Organic jams or jellies, with no added sugar
- Peanut or almond butter, organic
- Dark chocolate, minimum 60 percent cacao
- Teas (herbal, black, green, oolong) and/or coffee

❧ Eating Organic

The quality of our food is directly related to the health of our environment. No matter what your political party or personal beliefs are, there is a growing body of scientific evidence that indicates high levels of pesticide exposure during pregnancy and childhood can have lasting detrimental effects on a child's brain and behavior.

Two studies published in 2010, one in the *Journal of the American Medical Association* and the other in the *Journal of Pediatrics,* found that children with typical levels of pesticide exposure from eating commercially grown fruits and vegetables had a higher risk for developing attention deficit/hyperactivity disorder (ADHD), and children ages 8 to 15 with the highest levels of pesticide in their urine had twice the odds of having ADHD as those with less. This should make all parents think twice about what they feed their children. My advice is for pregnant women and children to limit the amount of pesticides in their diets, because from conception through 12 years old, the brain and central nervous system are most vulnerable.

Certified organic foods can cost more than conventionally grown produce, but the good news is that prices are coming down given the widespread and growing demand. To help consumers make informed decisions, the Environmental Working Group publishes an annual list of produce highest in pesticides, aptly named the Dirty Dozen; those lowest in pesticides are called the Clean Fifteen. The list changes from year to year, but apples, peaches, strawberries, blueberries, spinach, and lettuce usually make the "dirty" list, while onions, asparagus, avocados, eggplants, cantaloupes, watermelons, and grapefruits typically are "clean." My advice is, if you're on a budget, opt for organic if it's one of the Dirty Dozen and feel free to purchase conventionally grown produce on the Clean Fifteen list. Bookmark the website *(www .ewg.org/foodnews)* and print the list to take with you, so you can be an educated shopper.

Good Fats, Bad Fats

Fats are essential for providing the raw material needed to make hormones, the membranes that enclose trillions of cells, and for transporting the fat-soluble vitamins A, D, E, and K into the body. Instead of focusing on a low-fat diet, add healthier fats and limit those that aren't so good for you. Avoid trans fats—liquid vegetable oils that have had hydrogen atoms added to make them solid at room temperature—as they're bad for your heart. Many companies are removing

---

R℞ PRESCRIPTION FROM DR. LOW DOG
Go Organic on a Budget

According to the Environmental Working Group (*www.ewg .org/foodnews*), here are the 12 fruits and vegetables most likely to be contaminated—the "Dirty Dozen"—and the 15 likely to be lowest in pesticide contamination. Use these lists to decide when to go organic as your budget requires.

THE DIRTY DOZEN: Buy these organic
1. Apples
2. Celery
3. Strawberries
4. Peaches
5. Spinach
6. Nectarines (imported)
7. Grapes (imported)
8. Sweet bell peppers
9. Potatoes

10. Blueberries (domestic)
11. Lettuce
12. Kale/collard greens

THE CLEAN FIFTEEN: Lowest in pesticide

1. Onions
2. Sweet corn
3. Pineapples
4. Avocado
5. Asparagus
6. Sweet peas
7. Mangoes
8. Eggplant
9. Cantaloupe (domestic)
10. Kiwi
11. Cabbage
12. Watermelon
13. Sweet potatoes
14. Grapefruit
15. Mushrooms

---

them from their food products, and some jurisdictions, including New York City, have banned them altogether.

As to saturated fat, it's found primarily in meat, dairy (butter, whole milk), and palm oil. These should be consumed sparingly, accounting for no more than 7 percent of your daily calories. For someone who takes in 1,800 calories a day, no more than 126 calories should come from saturated fat. That's not much, so to make that mark, you need to limit red meat (10 to 14 oz or less a week), as well as foods made with whole milk, and chicken or other poultry with the skin on.

On the other hand, you want to emphasize healthy fats in your diet. Monounsaturated fat—found in avocados, nuts, seeds, olives, and olive oil—improve your cholesterol levels and may also improve blood sugar control, which makes them allies in reducing the risk of heart disease and diabetes. Have a small handful of walnuts or almonds as a snack and drizzle olive oil on salads and vegetables.

The polyunsaturated fats in vegetable-based oils have similar beneficial effects. One type of polyunsaturated fat—the omega-3 fatty acids found in fatty, cold-water fish, walnuts, and flax, hemp, and chia seeds—is particularly important for reducing inflammation in the body and the risk of heart disease (see the section on omega-3s for more information).

The bulk of my cooking is done using monounsaturated liquid vegetable oils. But there are a few things to keep in

R℞ PRESCRIPTION FROM DR. LOW DOG
Bean Bounty

In general, use four cups of water for every cup of dried beans (use less for lentils). Bring to a boil, then cover and simmer on low heat until they reach the desired tenderness. Black, adzuki, cannellini, kidney, pinto, and red beans all take about 1½ hours to cook. Check periodically to make sure there's still some water in the bottom of the pot as they simmer. If you have a pressure cooker, you can cook your beans in about one-third the time.

mind when buying, using, and storing them: Make sure to purchase only oils that have been naturally pressed, not those that have been extracted using solvents or high heat. When cooking with any oil, don't heat it to the smoking point, as it'll become carcinogenic. Smell the oil before using it to make sure it hasn't "gone off," or become rancid. To prevent rancidity, store oils in a cool, dark place.

There are many wonderful oils to choose from in the marketplace, based upon the style of foods you cook and your personal taste. I use grape seed oil when I want a neutral flavor and/or when cooking at higher temperatures. Lightly toasted, expeller-pressed sesame oil is fabulous in Asian-style cuisine. I use it in stir-fries, dips, and drizzled over rice. But the two must-have oils in any kitchen should be extra-virgin olive oil and organic, expeller-pressed canola oil.

Extra-virgin olive oil is pure, unprocessed, and unrefined and is the highest quality olive oil available. It's green in color, because it's loaded in polyphenol compounds that act as powerful anti-inflammatories and antioxidants in the body. Olives are generally low in pesticides, so you don't have to buy organic. Instead, you might want to invest in a less expensive olive oil for general daily use and a higher priced, delicious-tasting oil for dipping bread, drizzling on veggies, and making vinaigrettes.

Organic canola oil is a good source of omega-3 fatty acids and is the workhorse in the kitchen, as it can take a higher heat than olive oil and has a light flavor. You can use it in everything from sautéing vegetables to baking a cake. You may have seen some of the websites claiming that canola is harmful to your health, but this just isn't true. Many studies have been conducted on the health benefits of canola oil, and none have found credible evidence of harm to humans. In fact, in 2006, the U.S. Food and Drug Administration (FDA) granted canola oil a qualified health claim for its ability to reduce the risk of coronary heart disease when used in place of saturated fat in the diet. Some companies use hexane to extract the oil from rapeseed, so make sure you look for the words *expeller-pressed* on the label.

When I bake, I admit that I still use organic butter, as I like its flavor and consistency in certain sauces or when making piecrusts. But because it's high in saturated fat, I use it sparingly. There are also some margarines being produced now that are free of trans fats or hydrogenated fats. A number of them are quite tasty and make a good substitute for butter when you want the consistency of solid fat.

❧ Carbohydrates

There is a reason that carbohydrates have such a bad reputation. Look at where the vast majority of carbs come from in the American diet: white bread, soda, cookies, cakes, doughnuts, white potatoes, French fries, potato chips, white rice, white pasta, and sugar-laden breakfast cereals. Cheap calories people love to eat. Yet there is no question that these "empty" carbs are adding inches to our waistlines and wreaking havoc with our blood sugar.

For many years, we were told to "cut out the fat." Eating a low-fat diet was supposed to reduce heart disease and obesity. Well, many Americans have cut back on fat, yet we are still dying of heart disease, and more than 60 percent of us are overweight or obese. Now, we're told it's due to carbohydrates, and consequently, low-carb diets are the rage. But we should exercise caution before we go down the same road with carbs that we did with fats. We've learned that it was not so much the amount of fat as it was the *type* of fat we ate. I would make the same argument with carbohydrates. We've

PRESCRIPTION FROM DR. LOW DOG
Fats: Healthy to Unhealthy

BENEFICIAL FATS:
Polyunsaturated Fat
1. Seafood omega-3
   - Food sources: Salmon, shrimp, tuna, and other fatty fish
2. Plant omega-3
   - Food sources: Canola oil, flaxseed, walnuts, and leafy greens
3. Plant omega-6
   - Food sources: Corn oil, soybean oil, and sunflower oil

Monounsaturated Fat
   - Food sources: Peanut oil, olive oil

HARMFUL FATS:
Trans Fat
   - Food sources: Partially hydrogenated oil
Saturated Fat
   - Food sources: Beef fat, butter, and dairy fat

now moved beyond our understanding of carbohydrates as either "simple" or "complex" and are instead investigating how they impact blood sugar and insulin.

Since 1995, researchers at the University of Sydney in Australia have been evaluating thousands of foods to determine their glycemic index (GI). The GI is a number assigned to a food based upon how quickly it raises blood sugar in the body. You might also hear the term glycemic load (GL), which takes the glycemic index and then mathematically adjusts it to reflect the serving size of a food.

Foods with a high GI contain rapidly digested carbohydrates that produce a large and rapid rise and fall in blood sugar after eating. Fruit juice, potato chips, and candy bars all have a high GI. In contrast, foods with a low GI score cause a gradual, relatively low rise in blood sugar. An egg has less than 1 g of carbohydrate, and it has a very low GI/GL.

Why is this important? Well, when we eat foods with a high GI/GL, our pancreas must secrete insulin, the hormone that drives sugar (glucose) from the blood into the cell, where it is used for fuel. Insulin and insulin-related growth factors influence metabolism, cell division, and weight. If we continually eat a diet of high GI/GL foods, we will increase our weight, our cholesterol, and our risk for diabetes, cardiovascular disease, and certain cancers. This is in part because over years of rapidly rising and falling blood sugar, our cells become resistant to the effects of insulin. To compensate, the pancreas produces more insulin and insulin-like growth factors (IGF). This is the first step in the development of type 2 diabetes and heart disease. Studies also show that people with high levels of circulating IGF are at increased risk for developing colon, premenopausal breast, and aggressive prostate cancers. On the plus side, studies also show that eating a low GI/GL diet can improve blood sugar control, reduce the risk of heart disease, increase weight loss, and reduce body fat around the tummy.

The best way to eat a low GI/GL diet is to focus on getting your carbohydrates from fruits, vegetables, and whole grains. Skip the white bread, white potatoes, potato chips, white rice, and processed foods. When buying bread, read the ingredient list carefully. If it says whole grain on the front of the package, but it lists flours as multigrain, stoned wheat, organic, enriched, or unbleached wheat under the ingredients, you may actually be getting a processed, refined grain. Instead, you want to look for ingredients listed as whole wheat flour, whole oats, or whole rye. Pumpernickel is a great alternative to wheat bread, as it usually contains 80 to 90 percent hulled and cracked rye kernels. It has a GL of 6 (low is 1 to 10), versus a white bagel with a GL of 25 (high is anything 20 or higher). Choose bread that provides at least three grams of fiber a slice. At breakfast, have a whole grain breakfast cereal or a bowl of steel cut or old-fashioned Irish oatmeal. Add protein to your meals to lower the overall GI/GL of the meal.

R_X PRESCRIPTION FROM DR. LOW DOG
Recommended Reading

To learn more about eating a diet low in glycemic load, I recommend *The New Glucose Revolution* by Jennie Brand-Miller et al.

❧ Sweeteners

Each of us wants a little sweetness in our life, but our appetite for sweets has reached a very unhealthy level. Sugar consumption has increased from approximately 10 pounds a person per year in 1800, to 150 to 180 pounds a person per year in 2006. At the 2011 Nutrition and Health Conference, sponsored by the Arizona Center for Integrative Medicine, one of the most interesting and disturbing presentations was by Dr. Robert Lustig. A pediatric endocrinologist and obesity specialist at the University of California, San Francisco, he explained that the fructose in table sugar and high-fructose corn syrup, which are present in many processed foods and beverages, can only be broken down by the liver, using the

℞ PRESCRIPTION FROM DR. LOW DOG
My Favorite Cookbooks

- *The New Moosewood Cookbook*, by Mollie Katzen. I bought my first *Moosewood Cookbook* in 1979, and used it until the pages were stained and worn. Mollie has written a number of cookbooks, and all are excellent. If you want to start cooking healthy food, this is a great place to start!

- *Super Natural Cooking: Five Delicious Ways to Incorporate Whole and Natural Foods Into Your Cooking*, by Heidi Swanson. A beautiful writer, Heidi provides an inspired collection of recipes and detailed descriptions for how to incorporate natural foods into your life. Her vegetarian recipes are amazing.

same process it uses to break down alcohol. Like alcohol, fructose appears to dramatically increase the level of triglycerides, a kind of fat that circulates in our bloodstream and, in excess, can be detrimental to our health.

Our high sugar and HFCS consumption may be contributing to the rapid rise in diabetes, heart disease, obesity, and cancer. And this is in addition to the metabolic ill effects of fructose. The manner in which fructose is metabolized actually increases the sense of hunger and the storage of fat. Honey and agave nectar are also very high in fructose and are really no better than sugar. Although not all researchers agree with Dr. Lustig, I definitely left the lecture feeling that this is just one more reason to avoid processed foods, can the soft drinks, and limit the amount of other sugary foods I eat.

When my children were younger, one of the ways I dealt with the issue of sweets was a ritual we called Sunday Sundaes. I learned this from my Grandma Jessie, who would always make a special homemade dessert on Sundays after church—a strawberry-rhubarb pie, hot cookies fresh from the oven, or delicious spice cake. I kept the tradition alive, especially when my daughter was young, as she had a fierce sweet tooth.

On Friday, we would start planning what we would have for Sunday Sundae. It could be anything: cake, cookies, or pie. We would prepare it Sunday afternoon and have it with dinner. Whatever we made for dessert that night always tasted so good, and it was fun baking together. After we had our fill, I would either take the leftovers to the office the next day or throw them out on the compost pile.

Now before you accuse me of being wasteful, let me say that it just wasn't a good idea to keep a cake or pie around with only three people in the house. Otherwise, Sunday Sundae would've become Monday Sundae and Tuesday Sundae. Sweet desserts aren't for everyday—they're intended to be infrequent treats. Sliced apples and oranges, a bowl of dark red cherries, organic frozen grapes, or sliced cheese and almonds are more appropriate if you want to end your everyday meal with dessert.

There are a number of low-calorie or zero-calorie sweeteners in the marketplace, some natural and some artificial. Stevia, a plant native to Paraguay, has been used as a sweetening agent in South America for centuries. The FDA approved it as "generally recognized as safe" (GRAS) for use in natural sweeteners in 2008. Stevia has no calories and no carbohydrates and does not elevate blood glucose. I prefer the liquid stevia extract to the powder but must admit I haven't developed a taste for it in baked goods.

Xylitol, sorbitol, and erythritol are natural sweeteners made through a fermentation process of corn or sugar cane, and I prefer the taste of erythritol in baked goods to that of stevia. I typically advise patients to avoid aspartame, especially if they have migraines, seizures, ADHD, or autism. Sucralose (Splenda) seems a better choice if you want to have an occasional diet soda. I admit that I've never understood the appeal of sodas, whether regular or diet. Why not go for a cup of green tea, herbal tea, or water with some lemon or lime? Or how about a quarter cup of grape juice topped off with 6 to 8 oz of sparkling water?

❧ Protein

Our body uses protein to grow and repair itself. Unlike fats and carbohydrates, the body doesn't store protein efficiently, so we must consume it on a regular basis. If we stop eating protein, the body begins breaking down muscle within just a few days to meet its nutritional needs.

Protein-rich meals can also help boost mental alertness by raising levels of tyrosine, an amino acid that increases dopamine and norepinephrine in the brain. This is why eating protein for breakfast and lunch is important for enhancing your work and/or school performance.

So how much protein do we need? That depends on our age, body size, and level of activity. Nutritionists typically estimate our protein requirement by multiplying our body weight in pounds by 0.37. So if you weigh 150 pounds, you should be getting roughly 55 g each day of protein.

Most Americans get plenty of protein. Meat, poultry, fish, eggs, and dairy products, as well as plant sources such as soy, are considered "complete proteins," as they provide the nine amino acids that the body cannot make. However, vegetarians and vegans who eat a variety of whole grains, legumes, seeds, and nuts should have no problem getting adequate amounts of protein and the full complement of amino acids. The point for everyone is to get their protein from a variety of sources.

Fish is an excellent source of protein and is rich in omega-3 fatty acids. Wild Alaska salmon is low in mercury, high in omega-3s, and delicious. Farmed salmon is high in omega-3s but, because the fish are fed a diet rich in vegetable oils, it's also very high in arachidonic acid, a fatty acid that promotes inflammation in the body. I suggest you skip it. Shrimp, sardines, and canned light tuna are also good choices. Albacore tuna is higher in mercury, so it should be limited or avoided in your diet. Eating baked or broiled fish twice a week can reduce your risk of heart disease, but eating deep-fried or salted fish on a regular basis can actually increase your risk. Sorry—fish and chips are not part of a heart-healthy diet.

Although people immediately think of soybeans when it comes to protein, all beans are a great source of protein, as well as B vitamins, minerals, and fiber. Having been vegetarian for 12 years and being the mother of a strict vegetarian

R℞ PRESCRIPTION FROM DR. LOW DOG
Food Resources on the Internet

1. For organics on a budget: *www.ewg.org/foodnews*
2. For a glycemic index/load database for food: *www .glycemicindex.com*
3. For information on the Mediterranean diet: *www .oldwayspt.org*
4. For information on making healthy seafood choices, visit the Environmental Defense Fund at *www.edf.org/ oceans/*. Click on "Seafood Selector," where you can download a pocket guide.
5. For information on the safety and labeling of supplements, foods, and cosmetics, see the Center for Food Safety and Applied Nutrition (CFSAN): *www.health finder.gov/orgs/hr2504.htm.*

daughter, I have certainly cooked my share of edamame, tempeh, and tofu. While a small minority believes soy is dangerous because it contains compounds that can weakly bind to estrogen receptors in the body, the vast amount of research, even in women with breast cancer, shows that eating moderate amounts of soy is not only safe but is also healthy. Soy milk can be an excellent alternative to cow's milk. But soy chicken nuggets and soy burgers that contain highly processed soy protein isolates are junk food in my book. Remember: Eat whole foods as close to nature as possible!

Dried beans take a little while to cook but are so inexpensive. Make a pot on the weekend and you'll have some left over for burritos, red beans and rice, or a bean salad. I used to spend Sunday afternoons making bean burritos for my young son, so that I could pull one out of the freezer in the morning and pack it in his lunch. Having some canned beans in the cupboard is also a good idea for those meals when you're pressed for time. Just make sure they don't contain any disodium EDTA (used to maintain the bean's color), high-fructose corn syrup, or sugar. Also, because many cans are lined with bisphenol A, a chemical that can wreak havoc on our endocrine and reproductive systems, look for brands that identify their packaging as BPA-free.

Poultry products are also good sources of protein. The meat is low in saturated fat if you remove the skin. Choose white meat; dark meat is high in arachidonic acid. Skip the deep-fried and go for baked and broiled. As for eggs, a large one packs 6 g of protein, and contrary to popular opinion, having a few eggs each week is not bad for your health. Egg yolks do contain cholesterol; so if you have heart disease, use egg whites instead. Only buy poultry and eggs that are branded cage-free/free-range. Most commercially raised fowl spend their entire lives in tiny, dark, inhumane cages. I refuse to purchase eggs, chicken, or turkey that is not organic and cage free. Not only is this the right thing to do, but free-range fowl also tastes better, has a better fatty-acid profile, and has not been given antibiotics or growth hormones, which can adversely affect our health.

Red meats, which include beef, pork (no, it is *not* the other white meat), and lamb, are high in saturated fat, and an overwhelming body of evidence shows that excessive amounts

℞ PRESCRIPTION FROM DR. LOW DOG
Protein Content of Selected Foods

Tuna	6-oz can	40 g
Chicken breast	3.5 oz	30 g
Soybeans	1 cup cooked	29 g
Hamburger	4 oz	28 g
Salmon	3 oz	21 g
Lentils	1 cup cooked	18 g
Black beans	1 cup cooked	15 g
Tofu	5 oz firm	11 g
Milk	1 cup	8 g
Almonds	¼ cup	8 g
Soy milk	1 cup	7 g
Egg	1 large	6 g
Brown rice	1 cup cooked	5 g
Whole wheat bread	1 slice	3 g

can increase your risk for heart disease and colorectal cancer. The World Cancer Research Fund and American Institute for Cancer Research recommend limiting red meat consumption to no more than 18 oz a week and avoiding processed red meats that have been preserved by smoking, curing, salting, or adding chemical preservatives. Examples of processed red meats include sausage, bacon, ham, and lunch meats such as bologna, salami, and corned beef. Studies repeatedly show that diets high in red meats, particularly processed, are associated with an increased risk of colon cancer, whereas fish and skinless poultry are associated with a lower risk of developing the disease.

Being from Omaha, my husband loves steak. Humanely raised and infrequent, those are my only requests. A few times a year, I'll marinate a couple of rib eyes from beef that is grass fed and local, and he'll grill them. This satisfies his craving for red meat and my desire to keep him around a long time!

As to milk, people in many cultures of the world only consume milk during infancy. Because of this, many individuals, except those of European descent, have difficulty digesting lactose, the sugar in milk. Casein, a protein in milk, can cause problems for some people with allergies and autoimmune disorders. To make matters worse, the United States, Mexico, and South Africa are the only countries that allow dairy cows to be given bovine growth hormone to increase their milk production. Most countries have banned its use because it is inhumane and dramatically increases the need for antibiotics to treat the cows' swollen and infected udders. Although the growth hormone is inactive in humans, it causes large quantities of insulin-related growth factor to be released into the milk. The IGF in milk is not destroyed by pasteurization or by digestion. Remember, high levels of IGF have been associated with increased risk for breast, prostate, and colon cancers. If you're going to drink milk, opt for organic and limit your servings of milk and cheese to one to two a day. There are soy and nut milks readily available in the marketplace that provide protein and are free of hormones, lactose, and casein.

Last, when cattle are kept in overcrowded feedlots, they are given antibiotics to prevent infection. Of the antibiotics used in the United States, 71 percent are given to healthy livestock; only 8 percent are used to treat sick livestock. Although health care providers do overprescribe antibiotics, only 15 percent of all antibiotics in the United States are used to treat humans. Overuse of antibiotics leads to bacterial resistance to them, making treatments for common infections increasingly limited and, in some cases, nonexistent. More than 60,000 Americans die each year from antibiotic-resistant bacterial infections. One way we can turn the tide is by purchasing only meats that bear one of these symbols—USDA Organic, Certified Humane, or Food Alliance Certified. All of these symbols guarantee that the animals are not treated with antibiotics or given growth hormones.

My fervent hope is that we will all move to eating more plants and fewer animals and that the animals we do eat are allowed to live their lives in a humane manner. As the great 20th-century humanist Albert Schweitzer said, "Until he extends his circle of compassion to include all living things, man will not himself find peace."

Movement

〜

Lack of activity destroys the good condition of every human being, while movement and methodical physical exercise save it and preserve it.

—PLATO

As a teenager, I was fascinated with the history of ancient Greece, home of the Greek philosopher Plato, and the famous physician Hippocrates. Ancient Greeks placed a high value on physical fitness, believing that a healthy mind could only be housed within a healthy body. Some of the most beautiful statuary in the world is found in Greece, reflecting the classical Greeks' deep appreciation for the beauty of the physical form. The importance placed on health and fitness throughout Greek society was virtually unparalleled in history. Hippocrates, the renowned Greek physician, regularly prescribed daily exercise, moderation in food and drink, and ample sleep for his patients. Modern-day practitioners of preventive and integrative medicine are once again focusing on the therapeutic benefits of movement and moderation.

Those of us living today have the physical fitness of our ancestors to thank. Protecting one's band or tribe against nature's harsh elements, starvation, and the threat of attack by wild animals or unfriendly neighbors were all physically demanding. Though agriculture improved access to a steady food supply, early farming was highly labor-intensive, and in many early civilizations physical fitness was required by the state to ensure military and political strength. Yet today, according to 2009 Pentagon figures, roughly 35 percent of American men and women, aged 17 to 24, are unqualified for military service because of obesity, poor fitness, or other health issues. Wesley Clark, a retired U.S. Army general, described the lack of overall fitness in young Americans as a national security threat. As a physician, I see the lack of fitness and rising epidemic of obesity as a threat to our very survival.

Our technological success coupled with an abundance of high-calorie food is directly linked to our loss of fitness and high obesity rates. In the United States, even those of modest means have access to cars or public transportation, televisions, telephones, washing machines, indoor heating and plumbing, and food. This means we don't have to walk everywhere; go outside to play or talk to neighbors; wash and hang clothes by hand; chop wood for fires; carry well water in buckets to bathe, do dishes, or drink; plant, weed, and harvest our grains and vegetables; hunt or fish for food; or milk and tend our cows or goats. This dramatic decline in physical activity unfortunately has not coincided with a dramatic decline in caloric intake. This is in no small part why 60 percent of Americans are now overweight or obese.

Our bodies are designed for agility, flexibility, and strength, and our minds are designed for movement. The cerebellum is the part of our brain primarily responsible for the control and coordination of voluntary muscle movements and maintaining balance, posture, and equilibrium. Even though it seems effortless, movement is incredibly complex. For those of us who've cared for babies, we remember how hard it was at first for an infant to reach out and grab an object. With many attempts, as the months went by, the baby learned to roll over, sit up, crawl, and stand. The uncertain shaky steps of the toddler became increasingly coordinated until she or he was climbing up on the table and running down the aisle of the grocery store.

The magic of movement is coordination. To initiate and control our body's movements requires exquisite coordination of our muscles, nerves, motor cortex, brain stem, and cerebellum. For instance, to walk we must be able to contract all the muscles in our legs at specific intensities at specific times, while maintaining our balance on two feet. Our eyes, inner ear, spinal column, and cerebellum all work together to keep us from falling. The brain is constantly orienting our body position and contracting our muscles to counteract the effects of the Earth's gravity. It's interesting that astronauts, who can float while in space, lose muscle strength because no balance is needed in the absence of gravity.

As with many things in life, we often don't fully appreciate something until it's gone. When people damage certain parts of the brain or the nerves that travel along the spinal column, they can experience difficulty with movement and balance. You may have known someone who had difficulty moving an arm or leg after a stroke. Neurological conditions such as Parkinson's disease and multiple sclerosis can impair one's gait and coordination. Severe trauma to the head or spine, from a bad car accident, long fall, or combat, may result in paralysis.

Some physicians are specifically trained to address the needs of those with impaired movement. Physical medicine and rehabilitation physicians are nerve, muscle, bone, and brain experts who treat injury or illness nonsurgically to decrease pain and restore function. Physical therapists, acupuncturists, and massage therapists can also play an important role in recovery.

Like Hippocrates more than 2,000 years ago, increasing numbers of health care professionals are prescribing moderate daily exercise to their patients. According to the Centers for Disease Control and Prevention (CDC), regular physical activity performed most days of the week can reduce our risk of developing or dying from some of the leading causes of illness and death in the United States—diabetes, heart disease, high blood pressure, and breast and colon cancer.

Yet, the CDC also found that only 18.8 percent of adults 18 years old and older meet the daily recommendations for aerobic and muscle-strengthening activity! And the news is even grimmer for our children. A study published in the *Journal of School Health* in 2007 found that daily physical education was provided in only 3.8 percent of elementary schools, 7.9 percent of middle schools, and 2.1 percent of high schools in the United States. If healthy bodies are necessary for healthy minds, we are at risk of raising entire generations who have neither!

So how does exercise do all these things to improve our health? Physical activity lowers our risk for diabetes by enhancing the uptake of blood sugar by our skeletal muscles and lowering insulin resistance. It helps the heart muscle work more efficiently and stimulates the release of a chemical called nitric oxide, causing the blood vessels to dilate and reducing

PRESCRIPTION FROM DR. LOW DOG
Calorie Burner Chart

How many calories does physical activity use?

A 154-pound person will use up about the number of calories listed doing each activity below. Those who weigh more will use more calories, and those who weigh less will use fewer.

The calorie values listed include both calories used by the activity and the calories used for normal body functioning.

Moderate physical activities	1 hr.	30 min.
Hiking	370	185
Light gardening/yard work	330	165
Dancing	330	165
Bicycling (less than 10 miles an hour)	290	145
Walking (3½ miles an hour)	280	140
Weight lifting (general light workout)	220	110
Stretching	180	90
Vigorous physical activities	**1 hr.**	**30 min.**
Running/jogging (5 miles an hour)	590	295
Bicycling (greater than 10 miles an hour)	590	295
Swimming (slow freestyle laps)	510	255
Aerobics	480	240
Walking (4½ miles an hour)	460	230
Heavy yard work	440	220
Weight lifting (vigorous workout)	440	220

Source: *MyPyramid.gov*

blood pressure. Regular exercise lowers the body's levels of serum lipids and cholesterol. Initially, exercise increases the level of cortisol because our body views exercise as a stressor. However, over time our body becomes accustomed to the routine, and we essentially reset our stress response so that it takes greater levels of physical and emotional strain to increase our cortisol levels. This is why being physically fit helps us handle the ups and downs of life with more ease.

But we can overdo exercise as well. Some highly competitive athletes put tremendous stress on the body by overtraining, resulting in chronic elevations of cortisol. This can lead to osteoporosis, a well-documented problem in elite female athletes. The ancient Greek physician Galen said of the professional athletes of his time, "Athletes live a life quite contrary to the precepts of hygiene, and I regard their mode of living as a regime far more favorable to illness than to health." Even in exercise, moderation is key.

Exercise can definitely give you an edge against cancer, particularly of the breast and colon. According to the American Cancer Society, exercise may do this by reducing blood levels of insulin and insulin-like growth factors, which are associated with increased cell and tumor growth. As part of the Nurses' Health Study, researchers from Harvard University compared C-peptide levels, a marker for insulin, from the blood of 463 women who developed breast cancer to women who didn't develop breast cancer. Those with the highest C-peptide levels had a 70 percent greater chance of developing breast cancer compared with women with the lowest levels. C-peptide levels are also higher in women who are overweight or obese and aren't physically active. Being overweight or obese is an established risk factor for breast, uterine, and colon cancers. Exercise reduces the level of estrogen, a hormone that may increase the risk of breast cancer or make a malignancy grow larger and faster. And it reduces the risk of colon cancer, because it decreases the amount of time food spends in the intestinal tract, lessening contact between the lining of the colon and carcinogens found in food, particularly in red meat and processed red meats.

Being physically active is one of the best ways to maintain a healthy weight and healthy bones. Resistance, or strength, training is the only form of exercise that has been shown to slow and even reverse the decline in muscle mass and strength that can happen as we age. Resistance training increases bone mineral density, especially in postmenopausal women, which can help reduce your risk of osteoporosis. More muscle means you can burn energy more efficiently, helping you maintain your weight, and strong muscles reduce your risk of falling. Even just standing can burn a few extra calories and tone muscles, as you work to resist the effects of gravity!

Abdominal crunches, push-ups, and leg squats are resistance-training exercises that can be done without any special equipment; resistance bands are another inexpensive way to work out at home. Free weights and weight machines are excellent for strength training and are available both at gyms and for home use, but make sure you have a qualified instructor teach you how to use the equipment beforehand to prevent injury. Finally, yoga, Pilates, and tai chi can improve strength, flexibility, and balance, and they can be learned at any age. We gave my Grandma Jo a tai chi tape when she was in her early 80s, and she and her friends would follow along with

R̲X̲ PRESCRIPTION FROM DR. LOW DOG
Keep Moving

Physical activity includes exercise as well as other activities that involve bodily movement, such as playing, working, active transportation, house chores, and recreational activities. Here are additional ways to increase movement in your life:

- If you've been relatively sedentary, are over 50 years old, or have any underlying medical problems like heart disease or diabetes, ask your health care provider what kind and how much exercise is right for you.
- Remember, you can increase your level of physical activity by using the stairs instead of the elevator, parking farther away and walking, getting up from your desk every hour for a five-minute movement break, and doing more household chores.
- Listen to music that will motivate and energize you whether you're working out on the treadmill or raking leaves.
- Purchase a pedometer and gradually work up to 10,000 steps a day—roughly five miles. It makes tracking your movement easy. Having tried many, I like the Omron HJ-112, which costs under $25 and does everything I need. Many of my friends are in love with the Fitbit Ultra, which keeps track of your movement, calories, and sleep for about $100.
- Mix up your routine or try something new. Yoga, a blend of physical postures, stretching, and breathing

techniques, can improve flexibility, balance, strength, and relaxation. Try a local class or grab a DVD and practice at home. *A.M. and P.M. Yoga* by Rodney Yee is great for beginners.

■ If you're older and worried about your knees or flexibility, tai chi might be perfect. It's a series of slow graceful movements that improve flexibility, balance, and strength while soothing and calming the mind. Many health clubs, senior centers, and martial arts schools offer tai chi classes.

■ If you really think you don't have 30 minutes a day for physical activity, then break it up into three 10-minute sessions. Do yoga and stretching in the morning, go for a walk at lunch, and spend 10 minutes pushing the vacuum after dinner. Get moving—no excuses!

■ Invest in resistance bands. They'll help you tone your muscles, build strength, and burn fat. You can purchase them at most sporting goods stores for around $20.

■ Walking is one of the best ways to increase your physical activity. Get a good pair of walking shoes and alternate 5 minutes of brisk walking with 5 minutes at normal speed. Try working up to 60 minutes, or 10,000 steps every day.

---

the movements while watching it on the DVD player in the church basement.

The ancient Greeks were on to something when they said a healthy body was important for having a healthy mind. Even Thomas Jefferson understood the connection, saying, "Not less than two hours a day should be devoted to exercise, and the weather shall be little regarded. If the body is feeble, the mind will not be strong." I believe there is a direct correlation between the dramatic decline in physical activity and the rising rates of depression seen in many Western societies. Studies repeatedly show that regular physical activity reduces anxiety and depression and improves our psychological well-being. It does this in part by increasing the production of endorphins, our brain's feel-good chemicals, and increasing our tolerance to stress. Exercising outside is particularly helpful because exposure to natural daylight helps maintain our circadian rhythms, improving sleep. Going out for a walk gives us time to distance ourself from a problem and gain perspective on the situation. And I've always loved martial arts because it demands my complete and undivided attention. After an hour of working out, tension is gone and the world always looks brighter.

I'm fascinated by the growing body of evidence that shows regular physical activity helps preserve our brain function throughout life, and particularly as we age. After reviewing roughly 1,600 research papers, physicians from the Mayo Clinic concluded that aerobic exercise helps prevent dementia and cognitive impairment and that people who have dementia do better on cognitive tests after 6 to 12 months of exercise compared with sedentary controls. If you want to improve your memory, grab those walking shoes!

Researchers at Columbia University had healthy but fairly sedentary volunteers aged 21 to 45 (average age of 33) gently warm up for 5 minutes on a stationary bike or treadmill, stretch for 5 minutes, do 40 minutes of aerobic training (on a stationary bike, treadmill, stair-stepper, or elliptical machine), and then cool down and stretch for 10 minutes. Before and after three months of doing this exercise routine, participants took memory tests, aerobic fitness tests, and had an MRI scan of their brain. The results showed improvement on their memory scores and increased aerobic fitness and blood flow to the memory-related part of the brain.

There isn't a drug, vitamin, or pill that can come anywhere close to the power of physical activity for maintaining health. Exercise can extend your life—not just the number of years, but the quality of those years. It's never too late to start moving, as even small improvements in fitness can translate into real change. Some activity is better than none! No matter what your weight, the moment, yes the moment, you start adding more physical activity into your life, you'll begin to reap the benefits. Your heart will get stronger while your blood pressure, blood sugar, and insulin levels will gradually fall to healthier levels, and you'll feel fewer negative effects of stress. The more you do, the greater the health benefits and the better you'll feel. Physically and mentally, regular physical activity gives you the energy and confidence you need to get through life.

Vitamins and Minerals

Healing is a matter of time,
but it is sometimes also a matter of opportunity.
—HIPPOCRATES

For the past 25 years, I've been studying the role of dietary supplements in human health. I served as the elected chair for the nonprofit U.S. Pharmacopeia (USP) Dietary Supplements and Botanicals Expert Information Committee for ten years, beginning in 2000, and I now chair its safety subcommittee. The USP sets standards so that consumers can confidently expect a uniform, consistent quality when they buy and use prescription drugs, over-the-counter medicines, and dietary supplements.

I also teach both medical professionals and the public about the responsible use of dietary supplements. It is no surprise then that one of the questions I am frequently asked is, "So, doctor, what supplements do you take?" The list is actually pretty short.

I take a daily multivitamin/mineral (MVI), magnesium, and fish oil. I have a very good diet, but I know that I don't get all the nutrients I need every day, so taking an MVI just makes good sense to me. I take extra magnesium because it works like magic in preventing my migraines. The few times I have stopped taking it, I have had a migraine within a few days. It is inexpensive and safe, and it works. I take a fish oil supplement a few times a week, because I do not eat fish on a regular basis, and I am convinced that we need more omega-3 fatty acids than most of us currently get (the section on omega-3s will go into this in more detail).

Although eating a wholesome diet is always the best place to get the nutrients we need for our health, research repeatedly tells us that women do *not* get enough of what they need from their food. This can be the result of many things. Some women can't tolerate dairy products. Others may be vegan (they do not eat dairy, eggs, or animal products); vegetarian (no animal flesh); or have celiac, a digestive disease in which the body can't tolerate the gluten in grain.

Women also often need extra iron if they have heavy periods or when they are pregnant. Most of us need more vitamin D than we get from either the sun or our food. And medications can deplete certain nutrients. For instance, vitamins B_{12} and B_6 are lower in women taking oral contraceptives, and people taking proton pump inhibitors (Nexium, Prilosec, Prevacid) can become deficient in magnesium, iron, calcium, and vitamin B_{12} and can be at greater risk for bone fractures. For all these reasons, I recommend a multivitamin and possibly extra vitamin D as well.

All vitamins and minerals are necessary for health, but the following are some of the most important for women.

❦ Calcium

Calcium is the most abundant mineral in the human body and is critical for building and maintaining strong bones and teeth. Calcium is also needed for your heart, muscles, and nerves to function properly and for blood to clot. It can also lower the risk for osteoporosis and colon cancer, but you don't want to overdo calcium intake! It should be noted that some countries and researchers recommend far less calcium than we do in the United States.

For instance, in the United Kingdom, it is recommended that teenage girls receive 800 milligrams (mg) of calcium a day (versus 1,300 mg in United States), and adult women receive 700 mg a day (versus 1,000 mg in United States). The reasons for the differences are complicated and include the fact that there are growing concerns that high intakes of calcium may increase the risk for heart disease, kidney stones, and possibly ovarian cancer.

Because most multivitamins provide 200 to 350 mg a day of calcium, I generally tell women to try to get the rest of what they need from food. If you do need to supplement, calcium is better absorbed when taken in small doses (500 mg or less), and calcium citrate is one of the easiest forms to absorb.

Food sources: Yogurt, cheese, milk, fortified breakfast cereals, soy milk, tofu, sardines, salmon, and collard greens

Daily recommendations: Vitamin D enhances absorption of calcium, so it's usually best to take supplements that contain both calcium and vitamin D. Look for vitamin D_3 (cholecalciferol), which is considered more active than vitamin D_2 (ergocalciferol). The upper limit of calcium for women over the age of 50 is 2,000 mg a day from ALL sources. Do not exceed this dose unless under the supervision of a qualified health care practitioner.

- Girls aged 9 to 18: 1,300 mg
- Women aged 19 to 50: 1,000 mg
- Women 51 and older: 1,200 mg

- Pregnant and breast-feeding women: 1,000 to 1,300 mg, depending upon age

❧ Folic Acid

Folic acid is a B vitamin (B vitamins are water-soluble and help the body's cells metabolize). Sometimes called B_9, this vitamin helps maintain a healthy nervous system and is vital for protecting a developing fetus from birth defects primarily involving the neural tube. As the baby develops, the top part of this tube helps form the baby's brain, and the bottom part becomes the baby's spinal column.

Because folic acid prevents birth defects in these areas, a woman needs to start taking 400 micrograms (mcg) every day for at least one month before she becomes pregnant and then throughout her pregnancy. Unfortunately, 50 percent of pregnancies are unplanned, and studies show that only 27 percent of women are taking an MVI containing 400 mcg of folic acid when becoming pregnant.

Folic acid is also important in making new red blood cells, and a deficiency of it can lead to generalized fatigue and muscle weakness. Because of its importance to the nervous system, women who don't get enough folate (naturally occurring folic acid) in their diet can experience irritability, forgetfulness, mental fatigue, confusion, depression, and insomnia. This deficiency may also increase the risk of developing Alzheimer's disease in older women.

Certain medications and medical conditions might increase your need for folic acid. Talk to your health care provider if you have epilepsy, diabetes, asthma, Crohn's disease, celiac disease, autoimmune diseases (including rheumatoid arthritis and lupus), psoriasis, or chronic liver disease.

Food sources: Romaine lettuce, spinach, asparagus, turnip greens, broccoli, cauliflower, beets, beans, and fortified breakfast cereals

Daily recommendations: The upper tolerable limit is 1,000 mcg. You should not exceed this level unless under the supervision of a qualified health care professional.

- Adult women: 400 mcg
- Pregnant women: 600 mcg
- Breast-feeding women: 500 mcg

✿ Iodine

Iodine is necessary for the production of thyroid hormone. Your body can't make iodine, so you have to get it in your diet. Iodine deficiency can lead to enlargement of the thyroid and hypothyroidism.

Though we iodize our table salt, many women have cut back on their intake of salt to reduce their risk of cancer, high blood pressure, and heart disease. Perchlorate, a chemical in groundwater, blocks the uptake of iodine by the thyroid gland; in some states, levels of this chemical are high enough to cause iodine deficiency. This is concerning, as iodine deficiency is particularly dangerous during pregnancy, when there is greater loss of it in the urine. Deficiency in pregnant women can lead to miscarriage, stillbirth, preterm delivery, and such birth defects as mental retardation and problems with growth, hearing, and speech. Women who are breast-feeding their babies also have a much higher demand for iodine, requiring almost double the normal amount.

Food sources: Iodized table salt, saltwater fish, seaweed, shellfish, cow's milk, eggs, soy sauce, and soy milk

Daily recommendations: The American Thyroid Association has recommended that all pregnant and breast-feeding women in the United States and Canada take a prenatal multivitamin containing 150 mcg of iodine a day to reduce the risk of iodine deficiency. The upper tolerable limit is 600 mcg a day; higher doses should only be taken under the supervision of a qualified health care practitioner.

- Adult women: 150 mcg
- Pregnant women: 220 mcg
- Breast-feeding women: 290 mcg

❦ Iron

Iron is critically important to human health. Almost two-thirds of the iron in the body is in hemoglobin, the protein in red blood cells that carries oxygen to tissues. Iron deficiency is the most common nutrient deficiency in the United States, and the World Health Organization estimates that up to 80 percent of the world's population is iron deficient. Those at highest risk for deficiency are those with the highest need, including women of childbearing age, pregnant women, preterm and low-birth-weight infants, older infants and toddlers, and teenage girls. Several large studies have shown that babies with iron-deficiency anemia may have lifelong learning disabilities. Babies who are breast-fed generally have enough iron stored for the first four to six months of their life; after that, they may need iron supplements or iron-enriched cereals/formula.

Women lose an average of 15 to 20 mg of iron each month during menstruation, so they need a regular intake of iron-rich foods. Women who no longer have menstrual cycles due to menopause or hysterectomy only need 8 mg of iron a day. Iron deficiency can lead to fatigue, a decrease in work or school performance, difficulty maintaining body temperature, and more respiratory infections.

You might also need more iron if you have kidney failure, especially if you are on dialysis, or if you have Crohn's disease.

Food sources: Clams, oysters, meat, soybeans, kidney beans, lentils, breakfast cereals, blackstrap molasses, and spinach

Daily recommendations: Vitamin C enhances iron absorption from food and supplements. Also bear in mind that because iron is stored in the body and is difficult to excrete, toxicity can occur. Do NOT take more than 45 mg a day of elemental iron without supervision.

- Girls aged 9 to 13: 8 mg
- Girls aged 14 to 18: 15 mg
- Women aged 19 to 50: 18 mg
- Postmenopausal women and/or those 51 and older: 8 mg

- Pregnant women: 27 mg
- Breast-feeding women: 9 mg

❦ Magnesium

Magnesium helps maintain normal muscle and nerve function, keeps our heart rhythm steady and our bones strong, supports a healthy immune system, helps regulate blood sugar levels, promotes normal blood pressure, and can help prevent migraine headaches. It is also quite effective for reducing menstrual cramps. Wow, it's little wonder that magnesium is one of my favorite minerals!

However, studies show us that many of us don't get enough magnesium in our diet. This is further complicated by the fact that certain medications can really wipe out the magnesium we do get in food. The FDA has mandated a black-box warning that prescription proton pump inhibitors (Nexium, Prilosec, Prevacid) can cause magnesium deficiency, putting patients at risk for seizures and heart arrhythmias. Also, many diuretics that are used to treat high blood pressure deplete magnesium. Unfortunately, many physicians do not regularly check magnesium levels.

Food sources: Tree nuts, particularly almonds and cashews, brown rice, dark green vegetables, bananas, and fortified breakfast cereals

Daily recommendations: One of the main side effects of magnesium can be diarrhea and/or gastrointestinal (GI)

upset. If this occurs, look for supplements containing magnesium citrate or glycinate, as these forms are more GI-friendly. The dose shown beneficial for preventing migraines is 600 mg at night.

- Adolescents: 360 mg
- Adult women: 350 mg
- Pregnant women: 400 mg if 18 and under and 360 mg if 19 and older
- Breast-feeding women: 320 mg

PRESCRIPTION FROM DR. LOW DOG
Defining Vitamins

Vitamins are a group of substances that are essential for normal cell function, growth, and development. There are 13 essential vitamins—essential in that they are critical to the body's functioning:

- Vitamin A
- Vitamin C
- Vitamin D
- Vitamin E
- Vitamin K
- Vitamin B_1 (thiamine)
- Vitamin B_2 (riboflavin)
- Vitamin B_3 (niacin)
- Pantothenic acid
- Biotin
- Vitamin B_6
- Vitamin B_{12}
- Folate (folic acid)

Vitamins are grouped into two categories:

- Fat-soluble: Vitamins that are stored in the body's fatty tissue. The four fat-soluble vitamins are vitamins A, D, E, and K.
- Water-soluble: There are nine water-soluble vitamins. The body must use water-soluble vitamins right away. Any leftover water-soluble vitamins leave the body through the urine. Vitamin B_{12} is the only water-soluble vitamin that can be stored in the liver for many years.

❦ Vitamin A

Vitamin A has many roles in the body, but it's extremely important for vision. Vitamin A deficiency is the leading cause of blindness in the world, and the first sign of it is night blindness. This vitamin is also vital for the immune system, as it helps make white blood cells that fight off infections. Even a mild degree of vitamin A deficiency can increase a child's risk of respiratory and diarrheal disease and may decrease his or her ability to survive a serious illness. That's why the American Pediatrics Association cites vitamin A as one of the most critical vitamins during pregnancy and breast-feeding.

In the United States, vitamin A deficiency is relatively uncommon, but it can occur in people with persistent diarrhea (generally from Crohn's and celiac diseases and pancreatic disorders) and those with excessive alcohol consumption.

There are two primary forms of vitamin A. The most active, preformed vitamin A, comes from animal foods, especially liver and milk, and is absorbed in the form of retinol. The type found in fruits and vegetables is called provitamin A carotenoids, some of which can be converted to retinol in the body; the most efficiently converted, beta-carotene, comes from cooked or juiced carrots, peaches, and other orange-colored foods.

Although vitamin A is very important for our health, it's also important not to get too much preformed vitamin A; some research suggests that 5,000 international units (IU) a day consumed from food and/or supplements over a number of years can increase the possibility of bone fracture. This is especially noteworthy if you are at risk for or have osteo-porosis. Doses of more than 10,000 IU a day of preformed vitamin A during pregnancy have been shown to cause birth defects. My advice is this: Except possibly for breast-feeding women, do *not* take a multivitamin that contains more than 2,000 IU a day of preformed vitamin A, listed on the label as vitamin A palmitate or vitamin A acetate. There is no evi-dence that provitamin A carotenoids, such as beta-carotene, have any harmful effects.

Food sources: Preformed vitamin A—liver, milk, cheese, and fortified cereals; provitamin A carotenoids—colorful fruits and vegetables such as cooked or juiced carrots, canta-loupes, spinach, kale, apricots, mangoes, and peaches

Daily recommendations:
- Girls and women: 2,310 IU preformed vitamin A a day
- Pregnant women: 2,565 IU preformed vitamin A a day
- Breast-feeding women: 4,300 IU preformed vitamin A a day

❧ Vitamin B$_6$

Vitamin B$_6$ is needed by more than 100 enzymes in our body involved in the metabolism of protein; it's necessary for the production of hemoglobin, which carries oxygen within red blood cells; and it helps maintain healthy blood sugar and the immune system.

Animal studies show that a deficiency of B$_6$ decreases antibody production and suppresses the immune response. Vitamin B$_6$, along with folic acid and vitamin B$_{12}$, are important for the synthesis of neurotransmitters such as serotonin and dopamine—brain chemicals important for a healthy mood and healthy nerves—which may be why some research shows that B$_6$ can relieve depression in women with premenstrual syndrome. Vitamin B$_6$ is also widely used to alleviate morning sickness. Studies show that taking 25 mg three times a day reduces both nausea and vomiting.

Food sources: Potatoes, bananas, garbanzo beans, poultry, fish, oatmeal, fortified breakfast cereals, spinach, and avocados

Daily recommendations: The upper tolerable limit for vitamin B$_6$ is 100 mg a day; higher doses should be taken only under the supervision of a qualified health care practitioner. Prolonged use of higher doses can lead to irreversible nerve damage.

- Women 50 and younger: 1.3 mg
- Women 51 and older: 1.5 mg
- Pregnant women: 1.9 mg
- Breast-feeding women: 2.0 mg

❦ Vitamin B$_{12}$

Vitamin B$_{12}$ plays a critical role in the production of red blood cells; helps with the metabolism of proteins, carbohydrates, and fats; and allows your nerves to function properly. It's normally bound to the protein in food, but the acid in your stomach releases B$_{12}$ from the protein and allows it to bind to a substance called intrinsic factor. When this combination reaches the end of your small intestines, it is absorbed into the bloodstream. So, if you don't eat any animal products, don't make enough stomach acid, or take medications that shut down your stomach acid, you can't make intrinsic factor. If you have inflammation in your small intestine (Crohn's disease), then you can also have trouble getting enough vitamin B$_{12}$ to meet your needs.

Studies show that women who take oral contraceptives can become dramatically depleted in vitamin B$_{12}$, as can women

R$_X$ **PRESCRIPTION FROM DR. LOW DOG**
Digestible Vitamins

When I was a med student, I once saw an x-ray of a small pellet inside a patient's intestines. I pointed it out to the radiologist, and he told me that it was an undigested vitamin—enough said!

Here's a quick way to find out if your multivitamin will break down in your digestive tract: Put it in a glass of water (room temperature) and let it sit for 30 minutes. It should become a powdery-looking substance at the bottom of the glass. If not, it is time to look for a new brand.

who take the drug metformin (Glucophage), which is used to treat diabetes, insulin resistance, and polycystic ovary syndrome. Women who are trying to get pregnant need to ensure that they are getting enough vitamin B_{12}, as low levels are associated with miscarriage and possibly birth defects. People over the age of 50 have a harder time assimilating vitamin B_{12}, so the Institute of Medicine recommends getting it in the form of a dietary supplement and/or fortified foods.

Vitamin B_{12}, along with vitamin B_6 and folic acid, are all very important for mental health. Inadequate intake of these nutrients puts you at risk for depression. A large long-term study in Chicago found that low intake of vitamin B_{12} in people over the age of 65 was correlated with depression. Given that 20 percent of elderly people have marginal levels of vitamin B_{12}, I routinely order a vitamin B_{12} blood test every three to five years in all of my patients, starting at age 50.

Food sources: Chicken, meat, fish, eggs, dairy, and fortified breakfast cereals

Daily recommendations: Because there is a very low risk of toxicity associated with vitamin B_{12}, the Food and Nutrition Board have not set an upper tolerable limit. When high doses of vitamin B_{12} are given orally, only a small percentage can be absorbed, which may explain the low toxicity. Doses as high as 1,000 mcg a day have not been associated with side effects. Oral and sublingual preparations are as effective as B_{12} shots for the vast majority of individuals, but not for those with pernicious anemia, a condition that keeps the body from producing intrinsic factor.

If you are over 50, a vegan, or are taking a medication that can impair vitamin B$_{12}$ absorption, I suggest taking 500 mcg of vitamin B$_{12}$ a day, as studies show only 10 mcg is actually absorbed.

- Teens and adult women under 50: 2.4 mcg for adults
- Pregnant women: 2.6 mcg
- Breast-feeding women: 2.8 mcg

❦ Vitamin D

Like calcium, Vitamin D is important for maintaining healthy bones, as well as for optimal nerve and muscle function and for helping the immune system fight off infection. The beneficial effects of vitamin D start when we are still in the womb. Studies have shown that we have a lower risk for developing osteoporosis, and possibly type 1 diabetes and multiple sclerosis later in life if our mothers had adequate levels of vitamin D during pregnancy. It is hard for babies to get enough vitamin D in breast milk, so the American Academy of Pediatrics recommends supplementing with 400 IU every day.

Because we are busy building bones until our late 20s, it is very important for children and teens to get enough vitamin D. Later in life, as women go through menopause, vitamin D can slow the loss of bone density that occurs with declining levels of estrogen. There is a very large body of evidence showing that vitamin D significantly reduces the risk of falls and hip fractures in women over the age of 65. In addition to its effects on bone, mounting evidence suggests that vitamin D deficiency may be linked with insulin resistance, heart disease, depression, breast and colon cancer, and an increased risk for seasonal flu. Signs of vitamin D deficiency can include muscle pain, low energy and fatigue, moodiness, sleep irregularities, and weak bones.

Vitamin D is very difficult to get in your diet; most of it comes from exposure to the sun. However, if you live in a region above 40 degrees latitude (north of San Francisco, Denver, Indianapolis, and Philadelphia), the winter sunlight isn't strong enough to promote vitamin D formation. Wearing sunscreen also prevents the formation of vitamin D, though I continue to recommend the use of sunscreen, especially on the face and neck, to protect against skin cancer and skin damage.

For all these reasons, I recommend women take 1,000 to 2,000 IU of vitamin D every day, though in clinical practice I generally check everyone's vitamin D levels and then dose appropriately. It is shocking that even in the U.S. Southwest, where we have abundant sunshine, I see so many women who have very low vitamin D levels. I suggest you ask your health care provider to order a vitamin D blood test if you think you might be deficient. You should especially be tested if you don't get much sun exposure; have dark skin or a family history of osteoporosis, celiac, or Crohn's disease; or live in a northern climate.

Food sources: Sockeye salmon, mackerel, fortified milk, fortified orange juice, and egg yolk

Daily recommendations: The upper tolerable limit is 4,000 IU a day for anyone nine years and older. You should not exceed this level unless under the supervision of a qualified health care professional.

- Birth to 1 year: 400 IU
- Girls and women 1 to 70: 600 IU
- Women 71 and older: 800 IU
- Pregnant and breast-feeding women: 600 IU

❧ Multivitamins

As you can see from the previously listed vitamins and minerals, women need to make sure that they are getting enough nutrients in their diet. This is why I consider the multivitamin/mineral (MVI) to be the workhorse of nutritional supplements and the most important. The Centers for Disease Control and Prevention (CDC), which regularly monitors the nutritional status of children and adults across the United States, found that more than 75 percent of women do not get enough calcium in their diets, and more than 90 percent have inadequate intakes of folate and vitamin E from food sources alone! You still need to eat a well-balanced diet, but taking an MVI will fill in any nutritional gaps.

R℞ PRESCRIPTION FROM DR. LOW DOG
What to Look for in a Multivitamin

- In general, when shopping for a multivitamin, look for one that provides 75 to 150 percent of the daily value for vitamins A, B_1 (thiamine), B_2 (riboflavin), B_6, B_{12}, C, D, E, K, folic acid, and niacin, as well as the minerals zinc, copper, selenium, magnesium, manganese, and iodine.

- Do not purchase a multivitamin that contains more than 2,000 IU a day of preformed vitamin A, listed as vitamin A palmitate or acetate on the label, especially if you are over 50 or are at risk for or have osteoporosis.

- When possible, try to purchase a multivitamin that provides what you need in one to two pills; most of us don't want (or need) to take six vitamin pills a day.

- There is usually only 20 to 30 percent of the daily value for calcium in most multivitamins, because it is a very large compound and takes up a lot of space in a tablet. If you need more calcium, take it separately.

- Check the vitamin label for the United States Pharmacopoeia (USP) or NSF International (NSF) seals. The USP and NSF are nonprofit groups that verify whether companies offer contamination-free products and use good manufacturing practices.

- It is generally best to take your multivitamin with a meal that contains some fat to enhance absorption.

- To avoid possible interactions, take your multivitamin at least one hour before or two hours after any other medications.

Omega-3 Fatty Acids

◦◦◦

*Give a man a fish and you feed him for a day; teach a man
to fish and you feed him for a lifetime.*
—MAIMONIDES

I t seems everyone is talking about the importance of
omega-3 fatty acids these days. These are essential
polyunsaturated fatty acids that can't be made by
our bodies, so we have to get them in our diet.
There are three primary omega-3 fatty acids: eicosapentae-
noic acid (EPA), docosahexaenoic acid (DHA), and alpha-
linolenic acid (ALA). Plants, such as walnuts and selected
vegetable seed oils (flaxseed, canola, and soybean oils), contain ALA, but only a small amount of ALA is converted in the
body to EPA and DHA fatty acids. And EPA and DHA are
vitally important for our health. They come from fatty cold-
water fish, such as salmon, mackerel, halibut, sardines, tuna,
and herring, as well as from algae and krill. Unfortunately,
about one-third of Americans eat seafood only once a week,
and nearly half eat fish only occasionally or not at all.

Omega-3 fatty acids concentrate in the nervous system and
are critical for attention, memory, behavior, and mood. EPA
and DHA lower serum triglyceride levels; protect the heart
from potentially deadly heart rhythm disturbances; and lower
blood pressure and improve the function of blood vessels.

Increasing numbers of studies show they are beneficial for a wide range of conditions—depression, ADHD, joint pain, autoimmune disorders, and skin problems. This is, in part, because omega-3 fatty acids rev up the production of chemicals that turn down inflammation in the body. Inflammation is what drives many of the chronic diseases we are currently confronting, including arthritis, cardiovascular disease, metabolic syndrome, diabetes, and cancer. It's no wonder that the American Heart Association, the World Cancer Research Fund, and others recommend that we eat cold-water fatty fish two to three times a week. If that isn't possible or desired, take a fish oil supplement.

Independent laboratory testing of fish oil supplements sold in the United States repeatedly shows that they're free of mercury; however, levels of EPA and DHA are not always what they claim to be. You can go to Consumer Lab *(www .consumerlab.com)* or International Fish Oil Standards *(www .ifosprogram.com)* to check which brands are best for purity and quality. Fish oil supplements should be kept in your refrigerator or freezer and taken with a meal that contains some fat to aid absorption.

ᘛ During Pregnancy

Growing up, I ate a lot of fish. My grandparents went fishing all summer and would store their catch in the freezer. Catfish, perch, walleye, pike—these were regular staples and, of course, like most kids, I loved Mrs. Paul's fish sticks! Thankfully, I am blissfully ignorant of the cod liver oil I was given as a toddler. I find it interesting that even 40 to 50 years ago, people knew about the health benefits of fish—my grandmother always said it was "brain food"!

I became a vegetarian when I was 19 years old and, except on rare occasions, didn't eat meat or fish until 1994, when I was expecting my second child, my daughter. Given everything I know now, I wish I'd taken a fish oil supplement, especially while I was pregnant and breast-feeding my first child, my son. I had no idea how important these omega-3 fatty acids were to my own health or to the health of my child.

Supplementing with fish oil during pregnancy has been shown to lower the risk of premature birth and increase the baby's growth and birth weight by improving blood flow across the placenta. It may also help reduce the risk for postpartum depression. Omega-3 fatty acids, particularly DHA, are highly concentrated in the baby's brain and eyes, and it's vitally important that sufficient amounts are on board during the last trimester of pregnancy, when neurological development is very rapid. Studies show that babies born to women consuming fish or fish oil during pregnancy score better on tests that assess intelligence, attention, and visual acuity than those born to women with little omega-3 intake.

Fish offers other health benefits as well. In the medical journal *Clinical Review in Allergy and Immunology,* researchers reported that the majority of scientific studies show a reduction in the prevalence and severity of atopic dermatitis (eczema), hay fever, and asthma in babies born to women who took fish oil during pregnancy.

Here are a few more tips on taking omega-3 fatty oils during pregnancy:

- When you are pregnant, especially during the last trimester, eat low-mercury cold-water fish two to three times a week (see the chart on page 110) OR take a high-quality fish oil supplement that provides 200 to 400 mg DHA and 500 to 800 mg EPA a day.

- If you are vegetarian or vegan, there are DHA supplements made from algae available in the marketplace. However, to get DHA across the placenta and into the baby's circulation, you also need EPA, and there are no vegetarian EPA supplements currently available. This means you need to eat more plant-based omega-3 fatty acids in addition to taking your DHA. You can do this by adding a small handful of walnuts to your yogurt or salad, cooking with canola oil, or grinding some flaxseed and putting it in your cereal.

For Infants and Children

An ocean of evidence shows that DHA is vitally important for a healthy brain. Here's some food for thought: Omega-3 fatty acids, also called "smart fats," can help children focus and concentrate. A study conducted at the University of South Australia found that children with the lowest levels of DHA in their red blood cells had more learning difficulties, while those with higher levels had better reading skills and less anxiety.

This has been borne out in my own clinical experience, where countless numbers of parents have told me how fish oil, along with other sensible dietary and behavioral interventions, has helped their child with ADHD or autistic spectrum disorder. I have also seen many young children with eczema have an almost miraculous recovery when dairy was removed from the diet and fish oil was supplemented. Given all the potential upside, it just makes good sense to make sure your children get plenty of omega-3 fatty acids in their diet.

Here is more information on children and omega-3 fatty acids:

- If you are breast-feeding and eat fish or take fish oil, your baby should get enough DHA in your milk. If you cannot, or choose not to breast-feed, look for an organic infant formula that contains DHA and AA (arachidonic acid).

- Once your baby is weaned or is no longer on formula, make sure the baby's diet includes low-mercury, fatty cold-water fish two to three times a week, or consider supplementing with fish oil. There are numerous high-quality brands that make delicious liquids or chewable tablets.

- The Institute of Medicine recommends that children, starting at the age of one, get 1,200 mg a day of omega-3 fatty acids. I generally recommend giving a fish oil supplement that provides a daily dose of 300 to 400 mg DHA and 200 to 300 mg EPA.

For Teens and Adults

Omega-3 fatty acids not only help the way we look and feel, but they can also impact the way we think! Our need for omega-3 fatty acids is lifelong, so it's never too late to start getting more in our diet. Symptoms of omega-3 deficiency include fatigue, poor memory, dry skin, mood swings, depression, and heart problems. Although numerous things can cause these symptoms, the fact remains that the vast majority of us do not get enough of these important essential fatty acids.

The following are just a few reasons why we should consider adding more fish or fish oil to our diets:

Dementia. Many studies, though admittedly not all, suggest that eating fish and seafood might protect us from developing cognitive impairment or dementia as we age. Researchers at the University of California at San Diego found that elders with the highest blood levels of DHA have the lowest

R PRESCRIPTION FROM DR. LOW DOG
X How Much Fish Oil?

Look for products that are molecularly distilled and take with food.

For general health	Eat fish at least two to three times a week or take a fish oil supplement that provides 500 to 600 mg EPA and 200 to 400 mg DHA a day.
For skin health	Same as for general health, except in cases of psoriasis, when you should take 1,000 to 1,500 mg EPA and 600 to 1,200 mg DHA a day.
For eye health	Take a fish oil supplement that provides 500 mg DHA a day.
For prenatal health	Take a fish oil supplement that provides 200 to 350 mg DHA a day.
If you have heart disease	Take a fish oil supplement that provides 600 to 800 mg EPA and 300 to 500 mg DHA a day.
If you have high triglycerides	Take a fish oil supplement that provides 1,200 to 1,800 mg EPA and 800 to 1,400 mg DHA a day or talk to your health care provider about taking a prescription-strength fish oil.
If you experience depression	Take a fish oil supplement that provides 1,000 mg EPA and 400 to 600 mg DHA a day.
If you have menstrual cramps	Same as for general health.

risk of developing dementia. There's also evidence that when women take baby aspirin and fish oil together, they might have an added protective effect. Until we have more evidence, the dose recommendations for protecting the brain should be the same as those used to protect the heart.

Depression. Many factors are at play when it comes to mood and mental health. Diet is just one of those factors, and omega-3 fatty acids are just one aspect of diet. However, science shows that omega-3 fatty acid levels are connected to a variety of mental health issues, including stress, anxiety, depression, and bipolar disorder. This is in part because these fatty acids enhance communication among brain cells and help regulate mood by increasing levels of serotonin, a brain chemical that is often implicated in depression. A review of all the clinical studies examining the possible benefits of omega-3 fatty acids in mental health was published in the *Journal of Psychiatry.* The authors concluded that omega-3 fatty acids significantly improved symptoms in people diagnosed with bipolar disorder or depression, which in itself is a risk factor for heart disease. I'd say that there is enough evidence that, if you are struggling with either of these conditions, you should definitely consider fish oil supplements.

Heart health. According to the American Heart Association, "Omega-3 fatty acids benefit the heart of healthy people and those at high risk of—or who have—cardiovascular disease." That's pretty high praise from such a prestigious organization, and it's well deserved, given the extensive amount of research showing that omega-3 fatty acids decrease the risk of abnormal heartbeats, which can lead to sudden cardiac death; decrease triglyceride levels; and slow the growth of athero- sclerotic plaque (the stuff that clogs your arteries!). Heart dis- ease is the leading cause of death for women. In fact, more women die from heart disease every year than from all cancer deaths combined. In addition to regular exercise, adding fish or a fish oil supplement as part of a healthy diet is one of the most important things you can do to protect your heart.

Menstrual cramps. Menstrual cramps, also known as dysmen- orrhea, are caused by the release of inflammatory prostaglan- dins. Ibuprofen and aspirin inhibit these chemicals, which is why they work so well for cramps, but they also have side effects. More important, they don't get at the underlying cause of the problem—too much inflammation. Fish oil encour- ages the production of chemicals that quiet inflammation and reduce pain. Several studies have shown that taking fish oil for just three months can dramatically reduce menstrual cramping.

Skin health. All of us want healthy skin, and although using sunscreen is important, ensuring that you have enough essen- tial fatty acids in your diet is key to vibrant, hydrated skin. Omega-3 fatty acids reduce inflammation and redness of the skin when taken orally, which is why I always recommend them for women with dry, irritated skin, eczema, or psoriasis. A growing number of skin creams contain flaxseed, sea buck- thorn, chia, rose hips, and other plants rich in alpha-linolenic acid, the plant source of omega-3. These creams can improve the barrier function of skin, helping seal moisture in and keeping out pollutants that can dry and damage your skin.

The following are additional tips for omega-3 fatty acid intake:

- Do not take more than 1,500 mg EPA and 1,200 mg DHA a day without the advice of your health care provider or if you're taking medications that can increase your risk for bleeding.
- Doses larger than those mentioned under general health in "How Much Fish Oil?" on page 110 should be discontinued ten days prior to surgery to reduce risk for bleeding.
- Cod liver oil is not recommended for women over 40, as it tends to be quite high in preformed vitamin A, which may increase the risk for bone fractures.

❦ The Issue of Contaminants in Fish

Practically all fish contain some mercury and possibly other environmental contaminants such as dioxins, polychlorinated biphenyls (PCBs), or chlorinated pesticides,

R͟X PRESCRIPTION FROM DR. LOW DOG
Easy Fish Reference

To find out which fish are best to eat so as not to over-exploit the ocean's resources, you can go to the Monterey Bay Aquarium website—*www.montereybayaquarium.org*—and print the Seafood Watch pocket guide or get the app for your mobile phone.

which concentrate in fish fat. Mercury is particularly concerning as it can be dangerous to the brain and nervous system. This has led to a growing number of experts who recommend taking fish oil supplements that have all these chemicals removed as a safer option to eating fish. The greatest risk to health is exposure to these chemicals during pregnancy or early childhood. For women who are no longer able to get pregnant (for example, past menopause, have had a hysterectomy), the benefits of eating two to three servings of low-mercury fish a week, in my opinion, far outweigh the risks.

Mercury accumulates as you move from smaller creatures to larger predator fish. The level of mercury depends upon where the species live and on their size and lifespan. Mercury levels are generally highest in the large, long-lived predators (shark, swordfish, king mackerel, tilefish); intermediate in medium-size predators (trout, snapper); and lowest in short-lived (salmon) or smaller (shrimp, clams) species. This is why the U.S. FDA recommends that pregnant women and children avoid eating large predator fish and advises them to eat up to 12 oz (two average meals) a week of a variety of fish and shellfish that are lower in mercury (salmon, catfish, or shrimp). Use the following chart to learn about those fish that are safe to eat and those you should definitely avoid.

PRESCRIPTION FROM DR. LOW DOG
Seafood: Best and Worst

Preferred Seafood

According to the FDA and the Environmental Protection Agency, the following fish are lowest in mercury, meaning that they have less than 0.09 part per million. Enjoy these two to three times a week:

- Anchovies
- Butterfish
- Catfish
- Clam
- Crab, domestic
- Crawfish/crayfish
- Croaker, Atlantic
- Flounder
- Haddock, Atlantic
- Hake
- Herring
- Mackerel, North Atlantic, chub
- Mullet
- Oyster
- Perch, ocean
- Plaice
- Pollock
- Salmon, wild Alaskan
- Sardines
- Scallop
- Shad, American
- Shrimp
- Sole, Pacific
- Squid, calamari
- Tilapia
- Trout, freshwater
- Whitefish
- Whiting

Seafood to Limit

Eat no more than one to two servings a month of the following sea-food, as they are high in mercury, with 0.3 to 0.49 part per million:

- Bluefish
- Grouper
- Mackerel, Spanish, Gulf
- Sea bass, Chilean
- Tuna, canned albacore
- Tuna, yellowfin

Seafood to Avoid

Do not eat the following seafood, as they are highest in mercury, with more than 5 parts per million:

- Mackerel, king
- Marlin
- Orange roughy
- Shark
- Swordfish
- Tilefish
- Tuna, bigeye, ahi

Herbal Medicine

Much virtue in herbs, little in men.
—Benjamin Franklin

The history of herbal medicine is universal, having been used by all cultures and all peoples across the span of time. Fossil records date the human use of herbal medicine to at least the Middle Paleolithic, some 60,000 years ago. Already, our early ancestors were using their ingenuity to discover and effectively use plant medicines. In more recent centuries, botanical medicine has given birth to the sciences of botany, pharmacy, perfumery, and chemistry.

Today, with all of the advancements in modern medicine, it would be easy to dismiss herbal medicine as quaint, a discipline spoken of only in the past tense. However, in many parts of the world, including modern China, India, and many South American and African countries, plants have remained a primary source of medicine. And in the West, there has been a resurgence in herbal medicine due to an increasing dissatisfaction with the long-term, adverse effects of many of our modern pharmaceuticals. Because of consumer interest and demand, scientists are now actively engaged in studying the mechanisms by which plants heal, confirming many of the experiences and observations ancients made so long ago. I am delighted to have been part of this resurgence as both an herbalist and as a scientist.

I've been an *herbwyfe*—the old English term for a woman skilled in the art of herbal medicine—for more than 30 years. I opened my first herb shop in Las Cruces, New Mexico, in 1983 and spent many years making tinctures, syrups, ointments, and teas for my clients and customers. I learned from anyone who was willing to teach me: midwives, herbalists, *curanderas* (folk healers of Latin America), botanists, gardeners, grandfathers, grandmothers, and those who passed their knowledge down in books. I started teaching herb classes in my home in 1984, and by 1989, I was running a successful herb school. I witnessed firsthand the power of plants to heal as I cared for thousands of people before attending medical school.

After becoming a physician, I continued to use herbs in my practice, and I became increasingly interested in the research on plants for health. I served as the elected chair of the U.S. Pharmacopeia Dietary Supplements and Botanicals Expert Panel from 2000 to 2010, where my committee evaluated the

R
X

PRESCRIPTION FROM DR. LOW DOG

Recommended Reading

To learn more about how you can use herbal medicines safely and effectively in your own life, I highly recommend the *National Geographic Guide to Medicinal Herbs*, which I co-authored with friends and colleagues Rebecca Johnson, Steven Foster, and Dr. David Kiefer.

safety and effectiveness of herbal medicines and other dietary supplements. A key premise in integrative medicine, one that I have long shared, is that it's better to use mild remedies for minor health problems and save the more potent, and risky, prescription medications for more serious conditions. So when the evidence shows that St. John's wort is as effective as conventional medications for depression, that lemon balm can relieve anxiety, and ginger works for morning sickness, I generally start with those first.

I believe that everyone should have a basic knowledge of how to use herbal medicines, which is why I want to share a little of what I know about the healing power of plants with you. The following are just a few of the many herbs that I use for my own family and for the many patients I have cared for over the past 30 years.

❦ Ashwagandha *(Withania somnifera)*

For thousands of years, this herb has been treasured in India for its stress-protecting, or adaptogenic, effects. Its roots can boost immunity, ease anxiety, lift the mood, and enhance sleep. Indeed, its Latin species name, *somnifera*, means "to induce sleep." Ashwagandha is one of my favorite herbs for treating people with nervous tension that makes them feel on edge and irritable during the day, exhausted when it's time to go to bed, but wide awake when their head hits the pillow. Compounds in the roots bind to the same brain receptors that prescription tranquilizers do, but not as tightly. This means ashwagandha can calm and relieve tension without being habit-forming or overly sedating.

When people are stressed, they often get sick, especially with colds and upper respiratory infections. Here again, ashwagandha can help build resistance and ward off sickness. It does this by gently blunting the activity of cortisol, a potent stress hormone that turns down our immune system. In other words,

R℞ PRESCRIPTION FROM DR. LOW DOG
Calendula Ointment

- 1 cup dried calendula flowers
- Olive oil or almond oil to cover
- Beeswax (¼ oz grated beeswax per 4 oz strained oil)
- Tea tree essential oil (one drop per oz of strained oil)

Place herbs in a jar and cover with enough almond or olive oil so that there is one inch of liquid above the herbs and you can stir easily with a spoon. Put a lid on the jar and set it in a warm place for two weeks, shaking daily. After two weeks, strain the flowers from the oil, measure the desired amount of oil into a pan, and place on low heat. Add ¼ oz beeswax for every 4 oz of oil. After the beeswax has melted into the oil, test to ensure desired consistency by pouring a very small amount into a container and putting it in the refrigerator for five minutes until it hardens. If it is too soft, add a little more beeswax and recheck for hardening. Once you have the consistency you desire, add tea tree essential oil. Pour into salve containers and let harden. You now have a healing salve that can be applied (liberally) for diaper rash, skin irritations, cuts and abrasions, and eczema.

ashwagandha is an excellent choice if you're fed up with feeling sick, tired, and wired!

How to Use

Decoction: Simmer 1 tsp powdered ashwagandha in 8 oz of milk (cow, soy, or almond) for ten minutes. Add 1 tsp sugar and ⅛ tsp cardamom and stir. Drink in the evening to relax and unwind.

Dried herb: Take 1 to 6 g a day in two to three divided doses in capsules or tablets.

Tincture: Take 2 to 4 milliliters (mL) two to three times a day.

Standardized extract: Take 500 mg two to three times a day containing 2 to 5 percent withanolides.

Safety: Although ashwagandha is safe, avoid using it with prescription sedatives to prevent oversedation. Though it is sometimes used as a pregnancy tonic in India, it's probably best avoided during pregnancy because we don't have much scientific information on its true effects.

⚘ Calendula *(Calendula officinalis)*

I grow calendula in my garden, not only for the beauty of its warm orange blossoms but also because it is my go-to herb for minor skin problems. Calendula, also known as pot marigold, has long been a signature remedy for skin ailments, from eczema to diaper rash, from acne to abrasions. The German health authorities endorse the use of calendula for treating wounds, based on research that shows it is highly effective in helping wounds seal over with new tissue while also preventing bacterial infection. Studies also show that calendula creams can help prevent skin inflammation and irritation in women undergoing radiation treatment for breast cancer. I recommend calendula tincture as a mouthwash for mouth sores and to speed healing after tooth extraction.

How to Use

Mouthwash tincture: Put 3 mL in ¼ cup water and swish around mouth for 30 seconds three times a day as a mouthwash.

Topical: Creams and ointments are readily available, or you can make your own (see sidebar on page 120).

Safety: Use as directed. No safety concerns.

❦ Chamomile *(Matricaria recutita)*

Known in Spanish as *manzanilla,* which means "little apple," chamomile flowers smell wonderful and have long been used as a tea to ease colic and soothe fussy babies. The German health authorities recognize chamomile as an effective treatment for anyone suffering from gastrointestinal inflammation and spasm, such as irritable bowel syndrome, diarrhea, and heartburn. I often combine chamomile with herbs such as lemon balm or mint for a blend that calms as well as eases stomach and intestinal discomfort.

Chamomile, like calendula, is also one of my favorite herbs for skin complaints. A number of scientific studies have shown that chamomile creams and ointments relieve eczema as effectively as low-potency hydrocortisone, without any of the side effects that can come with using topical steroids. I recommend parents use topical chamomile for everyday care of eczema and save the steroids for more severe outbreaks.

How to Use

Infusion: Pour 1 cup boiling water over 1 tsp dried or 1 tbs fresh flowers and steep for five to seven minutes. Drink as desired. If making this for a baby, make sure the tea is room temperature and offer 1 oz *after* you breast-feed or give formula. This can be done two to four times a day. Make fresh daily.

Tincture: Take 3 to 5 mL two to three times a day.

Topical: Creams are available. Take as directed.

Safety: Although chamomile is generally very safe, extremely rare allergic reactions have been reported.

Chasteberry *(Vitex agnus-castus)*

Chasteberry is definitely a woman's ally. Sometimes called by the genus name, *Vitex,* this herb has been used for more than 2,000 years to treat problems associated with menstruation. Modern science confirms that it is highly effective for alleviating the symptoms of premenstrual syndrome (PMS) and breast tenderness, and for regulating menstrual cycles. It may also increase fertility in women.

Chasteberry normalizes fluctuating hormones, so it's a great remedy for women having irregular and/or heavy periods as they transition through menopause. I often use it for the same purpose in women who have irregular menstrual cycles after discontinuing birth control pills. When using chasteberry for PMS or irregular cycles, it should be taken every day of the month—not just before the menstrual period—and for at least three months to determine effectiveness; it's perfectly fine to take chasteberry for prolonged periods of time.

How to Use

Infusion: I'd pass on this; it doesn't taste very good.

Dried herb: Take 250 to 500 mg each morning in a capsule or tablet.

Tincture: Take 2 to 3 mL each morning.

Standardized extract: Take 20 to 40 mg each morning.

Safety: Chasteberry has excellent safety; however, it should be used in pregnancy only under the supervision of a qualified health care provider.

❦ Ginger (*Zingiber officinale*)

Ginger root—or more accurately, ginger rhizome (the underground stem)—has been prized in cooking and as a medicine for more than 4,000 years. Its Sanskrit name, *vishwabhesaj*, means "universal medicine," which signifies its effectiveness in treating many conditions. Ginger tea helps the body fight off a cold virus and soothe a sore throat, especially with a little honey; enhances circulation; and can warm you up fast on a chilly winter night. I often recommend it for women with Raynaud's, a condition where the hands and feet are unusually sensitive to cold. If you make a big batch of ginger tea, you can also use it as a compress on your abdomen to relieve menstrual cramps.

PRESCRIPTION FROM DR. LOW DOG
Many Ways to Use Herbs

Here are some of the ways you can take herbal medicines:

- Infusion: Steep 1 to 2 tsp of dried herb, or 2 to 4 tsp of fresh, in 1 cup near-boiling water for five to ten minutes. Strain and drink. Infusions are usually made from leaves and flowers of plants. Make fresh daily.
- Decoction: Simmer 1 tsp of herb in 1 cup water for five to ten minutes. Strain. Drink. Usually made from dried roots and bark of plants. Make fresh daily.
- Tincture: This requires an understanding of how to steep herbs in a blend of alcohol and water. Instructions for making tinctures can be found in many herb books and on websites. Tinctures are much more concentrated than infusions and decoctions and have a shelf life of at least several years. Sometimes vinegar or vegetable glycerine is used instead of alcohol, especially in products designed for children or for those who can't tolerate alcohol.
- Standardized extract: Commercially available in capsules or tablets and sometimes liquids, these concentrated extracts provide one or more constituents of the herb at a set and consistent level. Sometimes this constituent is highly important to the effectiveness of the herb; in other cases, it is a "marker" compound unique to the plant that helps ensure quality.

Most of our modern research has focused on the antiemetic, or nausea-relieving, properties of ginger. Studies confirm that it helps with the nausea and vomiting of pregnancy (morning sickness) and prevents motion sickness, because compounds in ginger stimulate digestion and the passage of food through the stomach. These compounds are concentrated by drying, which is why dried ginger is superior to fresh for nausea and stomach upset. Old-fashioned gingersnap cookies or candied ginger can be highly effective alternatives to tea and are often more convenient when traveling.

Finally, research is showing that concentrated ginger extracts can help reduce back pain and the pain caused by the inflammation of arthritis. However, these same studies show that many people get significant heartburn and stomach upset when taking large doses of ginger. The takeaway then is that a little ginger can relieve heartburn and nausea, while large doses can create both.

How to Use

Infusion: Pour 1 cup boiling water over ¼ to ½ tsp ginger powder and steep, covered, for ten minutes. Pour liquid off and discard powder residue. Drink 1 cup after meals for gas, bloating, or nausea.

Decoction: Cut an inch of fresh ginger rhizome into small pieces and simmer on low heat in 2 cups water for 15 minutes. Strain. Add honey and/or lemon if desired. Drink 1 to 3 cups a day for coughs, colds, sore throat, or to enhance blood circulation.

Dried herb: Take 250 to 500 mg dried ginger powder two to three times a day in capsules or tablets.

Standardized extracts: Concentrated extracts are typically used for arthritis. Use as directed.

Safety: Ginger is very safe in the amounts given previously, but pregnant women should not take more than 1,000 mg dried ginger a day, and people on anticoagulant medications (blood thinners) should not take concentrated extracts.

🌿 Lemon Balm *(Melissa officinalis)*

Once referred to as the gladdening herb, this gentle member of the mint family was revered for its medicinal properties by the ancient Greeks more than 2,000 years ago. It's a mild, effective natural tranquilizer and calming agent for the young and old and has been shown to relieve test anxiety in college students and agitation in people with Alzheimer's disease. I often gave it to my kids, usually blended with some chamomile and mint, to take the edge off a stress-filled day. European and German authorities also endorse the use of lemon balm for anxiety and poor sleep caused by tension and worry. I generally recommend a blend of lemon balm and two other sleep herbs—hops and valerian—before prescribing sleeping medication. There are no downsides to the herbs and plenty of problems with sleeping pills!

Like most members of the mint family, lemon balm is also a wonderful digestive aid, gently relaxing the gut muscles and easing gas, bloating, and indigestion. A study of 93 breast-fed babies with colic found a combination of lemon balm, fennel, and chamomile decreased crying time by more than half compared with babies receiving placebo over a period of

Milk Thistle for Your Liver

Some herbs have no Western drug counterpart. Milk thistle (*Silybum marianum*) is a classic example. Many studies show that it can prevent damage to the liver caused from environmental toxins, alcohol, and medications like acetaminophen. A study at Columbia University in children with acute lymphoblastic leukemia (ALL) found that milk thistle could reverse the liver toxicity that occurred as a result of chemotherapy, allowing children to receive all of their treatments on time. Milk thistle protects the liver without interfering with the effectiveness of medications, and there is no prescription drug that can do that. I recommend it to my patients who are taking statins, anticonvulsants, and other drugs that can harm the liver. The dose is 420 mg a day of an extract standardized to contain 80 percent silymarin.

---

a week. Scientists have also identified several compounds in the herb that are able to block the herpes simplex 1 virus, the virus that causes fever blisters or cold sores. Two clinical trials found that topical lemon balm extract shortened the duration and severity of oral herpes when applied three to four times a day. I always keep a tube on hand for those annoying and painful outbreaks.

The dried leaves steeped as a tea smell and taste delightful. I drink lemon balm tea, both iced and hot, regularly throughout the summer, making it from the fresh leaves growing in my garden.

How to Use

Infusion: Pour 1 cup boiling water over five to six fresh leaves or 1 tsp dried leaves and steep for five to seven minutes. Strain. Drink several times a day. If making this for a baby, make sure the tea is room temperature and offer 1 oz *after* you breast-feed or give formula. This can be done two to four times a day. Make fresh daily.

Tincture: Take 3 to 5 mL three times a day.

Ointment: Lemon balm ointments can be found at many health food stores and pharmacies. Apply as directed.

Safety: Lemon balm is quite safe and well tolerated by all ages.

❦ Peppermint *(Mentha piperita)*

Peppermint, along with other mints, takes center stage in my garden. I grow it in its own bed, as peppermint loves to spread out and has a tendency to take over if you're not careful. It's rare to find someone who doesn't enjoy the cool, fresh taste of peppermint or feel uplifted and lightened by its aromatic smell.

Mints have been cherished since ancient times for their ability to settle an upset stomach, support digestion, treat a cold, or ease a sore throat. The essential oils in these herbs—compounds like menthol that give peppermint its wonderful aroma—relax the muscles of the gastrointestinal tract while increasing the flow of bile from the gallbladder, helping the body more effectively digest fatty foods. That's why peppermint after-dinner liqueurs, like crème de menthe, have been so popular.

Scientific research has now shown that enteric-coated peppermint oil capsules are more effective than prescription medications for relieving irritable bowel syndrome (IBS). The enteric coating allows more peppermint oil to reach the intestine, where it reduces bloating and cramping. Because IBS is the most common GI complaint of young women, this is one remedy you want to remember.

I enjoy drinking a cup of warm mint tea when I catch a cold. It thins and loosens phlegm, acting as a natural and safe decongestant. I often make a peppermint compress to relieve sinus congestion and headaches. Mentholated lozenges for cough are great, FDA-approved, over-the-counter medicines. And last but not least, the versatile peppermint is often infused into topical rubs to ease the pain of sore muscles and arthritis.

How to Use

Infusion: Pour 1 cup near-boiling water over 1 tsp dried peppermint leaves or 6 to 8 fresh leaves. Steep for five minutes. Strain. Drink as desired after meals.

Compress: Pour 3 cups near-boiling water over 3 peppermint tea bags and steep, covered, for five to ten minutes. Remove tea bags and add 1 cup ice cubes. Dip washcloth into cold tea and apply to forehead to relieve sinus or tension headache.

Enteric-coated peppermint oil: Take 0.2 mL peppermint oil two to three times a day before meals for intestinal cramping or irritable bowel syndrome.

Lozenges: For sore throat and cough, lozenges should contain 5 to 10 mg menthol; children two and under should not use these.

Topical: Many mentholated ointments are available on the market. Apply two to three times a day as needed.

Safety: Peppermint tea is quite safe but may worsen heartburn in people who have gastroesophageal reflux disease (GERD). Do not apply peppermint oil to the face of an infant or child under the age of five, as it can cause spasms that impair breathing.

🌿 Rhodiola *(Rhodiola rosea)*

Rhodiola, sometimes referred to as Arctic or golden root, grows at high altitudes in Europe and Asia and has been used in traditional medicine in Russia and in Scandinavian countries for centuries. It has been credited with easing depression, decreasing fatigue, and preventing high-altitude sickness—the Vikings relied on it for enhancing mental and physical endurance during their long travels. It remains popular in Sweden and other Scandinavian countries as a rejuvenating tonic.

I became fascinated with rhodiola in 1998, after hearing a psychiatrist at Columbia University speak about his experience using it to treat depression. Over the years, I have found that it can indeed help depression as well as dramatically improve the quality of life for those living with fibromyalgia and/or chronic fatigue. A number of clinical studies have confirmed its antidepressant activity, as well as its ability to improve sleep, lessen pain, and boost energy in people with chronic fatigue. Researchers at the University of California in Los Angeles (UCLA) have also shown that rhodiola alleviates anxiety. It's little wonder that rhodiola is one of my favorite herbs.

How to Use

Standardized extract: The dose used in clinical trials ranged from 200 to 680 mg a day of extracts standardized to 3 to 5 percent rosavin and 0.8 to 1.0 percent salidroside (two active compounds found in the root). I generally start with 100 to 200 mg a day for one to two weeks and then gradually increase by 100 mg each week as needed. Most people have good success with doses of 300 to 500 mg a day taken in two divided doses. In the case of rhodiola, I would purchase standardized extracts to ensure you're getting what you pay for.

❦ Sage *(Salvia officinalis)*

The genus name *Salvia* is from the word *salvere,* "to save" or "to heal," likely given in honor of sage's long history as a medicine. The Greeks and Romans revered the herb, as it was said to clear the mind and impart wisdom, hence the term *sage* being associated with a wise elder. Interestingly, there may be something to this relationship between sage and the mind. Researchers have found that compounds in sage inhibit acetylcholinesterase, an enzyme implicated in dementia. Animal studies and human clinical trials suggest that sage may improve mood and mental clarity in both healthy adults and those with Alzheimer's dementia.

Sage is also a very old remedy for excessive sweating, a fact that I took to heart as I transitioned through menopause. Although I had recommended sage for years, it was far more meaningful to experience how well it worked firsthand. Not only did the sage tea relieve my hot flashes, it also made me feel calm and alert. I often combine sage with other herbs such as shatavari, chasteberry, hops, or black cohosh for menopausal symptoms, but it is also quite effective when used alone.

My grandmother used to give me sage tea and salt as a gargle when I had a sore throat. It always worked great, and I have used it with my own children as well as countless patients. Science has now confirmed what my grandmother already knew. A clinical trial of 286 people with acute pharyngitis (sore throat) found that a 15 percent sage spray was superior to a placebo spray for relieving symptoms, and symptom relief occurred within two hours of the first treatment! Similar results were found when an echinacea/sage spray was compared with a conventional analgesic spray in 154 people with acute sore throat. Not only does sage relieve the pain but it also helps to fight the infection.

How to Use

Infusion: Steep 1 tsp chopped sage in 1 cup water for ten minutes. Strain. Drink or use as a gargle for sore throat.

Dried herb: Take 500 mg dried sage leaf two times a day in capsule or tablet form.

Tincture: Take 2 mL tincture two times a day, or per manufacturer's recommendation. You can add 5 mL of tincture to 1 cup water and use as a gargle three times a day.

Safety: Sage leaf is safe in cooking and when used in the recommended doses. However, the essential oil of sage, often used in aromatherapy, contains thujone, which can be harmful if taken in quantity. For this reason, I recommend avoiding any internal use of sage essential oil. Sage gargles are safe for anyone; however, pregnant women should not use medicinal-strength doses of sage internally.

🌿 Shatavari *(Asparagus racemosus)*

In Sanskrit, *shatavari* means "she who possesses one hundred husbands," a strong indication of the value placed on the rejuvenating properties of this plant. Prepared from the roots of the wild asparagus, a relative of the common asparagus that so many of us love to eat, shatavari has been used in the traditional medicine of India for more than 4,000 years. It is said to act as a tonic to the female reproductive organs, bringing about harmony, especially during times of stress or illness. It was commonly used to enhance breast milk production, aid fertility, and ease menopause-related symptoms.

I think of shatavari as an herb for women in transition. Among the traditional healers of India, it is considered a *sattvic* herb, meaning that it helps bring the mind and emotions into balance while encouraging feelings of love and devotion. I share this when I recommend the herb to a woman and encourage her to be open to that experience when taking it—open to the idea of balance, harmony, and receptivity to feelings of love for both self and others.

I often recommend that a new mother take shatavari for four to six weeks after giving birth as a way to strengthen her and ensure a good supply of breast milk. But I also tell her that tradition holds that shatavari will open her heart, so that she may fall deeply in love with her child. For a woman transitioning through menopause, I highly recommend it to ease hot flashes and night sweats so that she feels more rested and centered, but shatavari can also help her fall in love with her changing self. I believe that this is why it has the reputation as an aphrodisiac for women: When we are in balance and centered, the love flows more freely from and to us.

R℞ PRESCRIPTION FROM DR. LOW DOG
Take Tea

Note: To get the most benefit from tea, don't add sugar, milk, or cream.

All tea types come from the same plant leaf (*Camillia sinensis*), but are distinguished by the type of processing they undergo.

- White tea: Made with younger leaves and buds that have been very lightly withered in the sun to allow a small amount of oxidation and then baked dry
- Green tea: Made by immediately applying heat (steaming or dry cooking) to the leaves after harvest to prevent oxidation; the most studied tea for its health benefits
- Oolong tea: Made with semi-oxidized leaves (between green and black teas)
- Black tea: Made with leaves that are allowed to wither in the sun, then bruised or cut to release the leaf juices and enzymes until they are completely oxidized and then dried; has the highest caffeine content (Tieraona's favorite morning tea)

How to Use

Decoction: Simmer 1 tsp dried root in 1 cup milk (soy, almond, or cow) for 10 to 15 minutes. Strain. Add $^1/_8$ tsp cardamom and 1 tsp sugar. Drink 1 to 2 cups a day.

Dried herb: Take 500 mg one to two times a day in capsule or tablet form.

Tincture: Take 2 to 3 mL two to three times a day.

Safety: Shatavari is quite safe, although there is insufficient information to determine its safety in pregnancy.

❦ Tea *(Camellia sinensis)*

White, green, oolong, and black tea all come from the same plant. They just undergo different processing. The least processed is white tea, which is rich in antioxidant polyphenol compounds, called catechins. Then comes the more popular green tea, in which the leaves are harvested, steamed, and cooled to prevent oxidation. After cooling, the leaves are pressed and rolled while being gently dried with hot air. In contrast, black tea is allowed to wither, oxidize, and ferment, which explains its color. It is higher in caffeine and lower in antioxidant compounds but, unlike green tea, it maintains its flavor for years. Oolong tea falls right between green and black tea. Green tea is widely consumed in Asian countries, whereas black tea is preferred in Europe and North America.

Science has definitely shown that drinking tea, especially green tea, is good for your health. For instance, a large study found that women who drank two to three cups of tea a day had a lower risk of heart disease, while a study in men found that those who drank green tea had lower cholesterol levels. Overall, I would say that green tea helps protect your cardiovascular system. Some studies have shown that green and oolong teas can help somewhat with weight loss because they boost metabolism and help burn fat. Don't expect miracles, but drinking a cup of tea before meals might be a very useful part of a weight management strategy. Tea may also help protect against certain cancers, such as oral and skin cancers, though the evidence is less clear.

I often wondered why I, like so many others, felt a sense of calm alertness after drinking a cup of tea. Tea contains caffeine, and caffeine generally makes me jittery. I recently learned, though, that tea also contains L-theanine, an amino acid that has a quieting effect on the nervous system. In Japan, it's used to treat anxiety, and it's gaining popularity as a dietary supplement in the United States. The combination of L-theanine and caffeine makes tea an ideal beverage if you need to focus on work or studies but don't like the side effects of too much coffee.

Because caffeine is rapidly soluble in water, if you want to make your own decaf, simply steep your tea for about 30 seconds, throw out the water, and pour fresh hot water over the leaves and allow to steep. Although you'll lose some of the catechins, you can enjoy a cup of tea in the afternoon without having to buy decaf. But if you want to get the health benefits of tea, skip the instant varieties, as well as the premade teas in a bottle, as they are very low in the tea catechins that help your body repair itself and protect against environmental damage.

How to Use

Infusion: Bring 1 cup water to a boil, let sit for about 30 to 60 seconds, and then pour over 1 tsp loose tea leaves or high-quality tea in a tea bag. Steep for about two minutes. Don't steep too long or it will taste bitter. Drink 1 to 3 cups a day. If you don't care for green tea, start with black and then move to oolong. Over time, you will gradually develop a taste for the green variety.

Standardized extracts: Green tea extracts are available that are standardized to catechins, particularly epigallocatechin-3-gallate, or EGCG. The dose is generally 500 mg one to two times a day.

Safety: There are really no safety problems associated with tea, but pregnant women are cautioned to limit caffeine and should stick with 2 to 3 cups a day. There have been a few rare reports of liver damage associated with taking concentrated green tea extracts that contain 500 mg or more of EGCG. To avoid the risk, make sure to take with food.

Sleep

*A good laugh and a long sleep
are the best cures in the doctor's book.*
—Irish proverb

By the time we turn 50, we've spent roughly 16 years, or a third of our lives, asleep. I figure that 16 years of doing anything should give us some expertise! Yet sleep has proved an elusive companion for much of my life. From waking to nurse my babies, staying up for births as a midwife and physician, being on call at the hospital, and frequently traveling across time zones, I have spent many years getting by on six hours of shut-eye, sleeping deeply until around 3 or 4 a.m. and then not being able to go back to sleep. I admit I am occasionally envious of my husband, children, and others who drift off to sleep the moment their heads hit the pillow for eight blissful hours of uninterrupted slumber.

Tonight, and every night, there'll be roughly 70 million Americans, who, like me, will be struggling to fall asleep or stay asleep, according to the National Sleep Foundation. We toss and turn, fluff our pillows, take an herbal remedy or prescription sleeping pill, and pray for the sandman to visit. We all know that when we don't get enough sleep, we feel tired and sleepy, making it hard for us to respond rapidly to changing situations or make sound judgments.

Here are some sobering facts: Seventeen hours of sustained wakefulness leads to a decrease in performance equivalent to a blood alcohol level of 0.05 percent, the same as drinking two glasses of wine. The National Highway Traffic Safety Administration estimates there are 56,000 sleep-related road crashes annually in the United States, resulting in 40,000 injuries and 1,550 fatalities. Inadequate rest also puts tremendous stress on the body, which explains in part why scientists have linked chronic insomnia with diabetes, heart disease, depressed mood, and possibly breast and colon cancer. For those struggling with weight, research shows that sleep loss increases the risk of obesity because body chemicals involved in controlling appetite and weight gain are released during sleep. As if we didn't have enough things to worry about while we're lying there, trying to sleep!

We can control several things that can help us sleep. One is light—or more precisely, the timing and type of light we're exposed to in our sleep. When our eyes are exposed to sunlight, we feel alert and awake because melatonin, the hormone of darkness, is suppressed. As nighttime falls, melatonin is secreted by the pineal gland to prepare us for sleep. Traditionally, humans would go to sleep one to two hours after nightfall and wake up with the sun. The red light from fire, which lit our dark nights for thousands of years, had no effect on melatonin, but the blue wavelengths from daytime sunlight (they're the reason the sky looks blue) suppress melatonin, as does the blue light from televisions, lamps, computer screens, and many bedside digital clocks. This is why it's so important to simulate nightfall in your home by putting dimmer switches on lights and lamps and installing a free software called F.lux on your computer, which changes the light on the screen from blue during the day to a warmer red at night, so it won't interfere with your sleep.

The almost surreal busyness of modern life also affects sleep. From sunrise to way beyond sunset, we're running all the time, whether we're working inside the home, outside the home, or both. Managing children, shopping, cooking, working, cleaning, paying bills, handling relationships, exercising, and being plugged into technology 24/7 can't help but have an impact on sleep. We can't expect to run around until 9:30 p.m., drink a cup of chamomile tea or take a sleeping pill, and think we'll drift off into a peaceful slumber 30 minutes later—especially if we're watching TV, checking email, or answering texts until 9:50! If we want to sleep well, we have to create some nightly rituals to prepare our mind and body for rest, like the ones listed in the sidebar "Getting Ready for Sleep."

Although various sleep strategies are extremely helpful for getting a good night's sleep, it's important to accept that sometimes we aren't going to sleep well and that our sleep patterns may change as we transition through different phases of our life.

Shortly after I moved to our ranch east of Santa Fe, I noticed a change in my sleep patterns. I'd fall asleep around 9 p.m., and sleep deeply until around 1 a.m. After a few nights of lying restlessly awake in bed, I started getting up to write or read until around 3 a.m., when I'd get tired, go back to bed, and sleep until 6 a.m. I couldn't believe I was having so much trouble sleeping. I set the thermostat at 65°F, the optimal temperature for sleep, meditated, eliminated all caffeine and alcohol, listened to CDs of ocean waves, did guided imagery and breathing exercises, took melatonin, and tried tinctures of California poppy and hops. And still I'd wake up every morning between 1 and 2 a.m. A friend thought it was connected to a past life. Well intentioned, I'm sure, but that didn't ring true. Another friend who practices homeopathy gave me a homeopathic remedy. Didn't work. An acupuncturist colleague told me waking at this particular time was due to an imbalance in my liver energy. The bitter herbs he prescribed did nothing to help me sleep.

I began to dread going to bed. Then, quite by accident, I stumbled upon a book by A. Roger Ekirch, a history professor at Virginia Tech, entitled *At Day's Close: Night in Times Past*. His research suggested that people didn't traditionally sleep the whole night through. Before electricity was widely available, people typically slept in two distinct periods they referred to as first sleep and second sleep. Within an hour or two after sunset, people went to bed and slept around four hours. They would wake up for a couple of hours and make love, get up and do chores, visit with family members, or quietly reflect upon their dreams, until returning to bed about 2 a.m. and sleeping until sunrise.

Ekirch's book made me wonder if being out in the garden and riding horses all day, and then being immersed in almost complete darkness at night, had reset my internal clock. Maybe I didn't have insomnia, a rotten past life, or a faulty liver after all. Maybe it wasn't natural anymore for me to sleep an uninterrupted eight hours. Being awake for brief periods during the night hadn't left me feeling tired. On the contrary, most days I greeted the morning rested, and during the wee hours of the night, I welcomed a deeper, more creative part of myself.

What I'm trying to say is that it's important to think of nighttime as a period of rest and tranquility rather than as a battle to be waged between our waking and sleeping selves. It can be incredibly freeing simply to accept that our sleep cycles vary and that there will be nights when we don't sleep well. Now when I can't sleep, I decide whether to get up and write or read or to meditate and focus on my breathing. I don't toss and turn all night, frustrated that I'm not sleeping. I trust that my body will get the respite it needs, as long as I create the space for it to occur. I don't say I'm a poor sleeper. When someone asks how I slept, I say, "I rested." Like many things in life, the way we look at sleep determines how it affects us. When we think about night as a time of quiet and calm, instead of only as a time for sleep, we can actually create a more relaxed space for sleep to occur.

R̶X PRESCRIPTION FROM DR. LOW DOG
Getting Ready for Sleep

The following are some things you can adapt to your own life and schedule (if you have children, you can alter this routine so they can join you, or add other rituals, like bedtime stories, that relax the kids and you):

- Around two hours before bedtime, start dimming the lights in your living space and shutting down your computer, cell phone, television, and anything else emitting blue light.
- A half hour later, spend 10 minutes writing down any

"to-do" items for the following day in a notebook you keep by the bed. This is so you don't have to think about, or try to remember, them during the night.

■ Now prepare a warm bath with fragrant essential oils like neroli, sandalwood, chamomile, or lavender.

■ Soak by candlelight for about 20 minutes.

■ By this time, the lights should be very dim, and all television and communication devices completely shut off.

■ In comfy sleeping clothes, spend ten minutes doing some gentle stretching.

■ Mist your pillows and sheets with lavender or jasmine essential oil. You can make your own by combining ten drops of essential oil with 2 oz of water in a glass bottle with a spray pump.

■ Turn on soft music or white noise and slide into bed. Think about one person or event that happened during the day for which you're grateful. Take a few deep, slow breaths, and invite sleep into your night.

❦ Common Causes of Insomnia

If you've been having difficulty falling or staying asleep, it's a good idea to schedule a talk with your health care provider to rule out any underlying medical cause, such as the following:

Sleep apnea. A fairly common condition that causes pauses in breathing or shallow breaths while sleeping. People with the condition often snore, snort, and gasp throughout the night, and because they repeatedly move from deep to light sleep, they feel exhausted during the day. Your health care professional can order a sleep study if you think you have sleep apnea, or you can suggest one to your partner if his/her snoring is keeping you up!

Restless leg syndrome (RLS). A neurological condition characterized by unpleasant sensations of crawling, creeping, or pulling in the legs and an overwhelming need to move them, particularly when lying down to relax, RLS affects roughly one in ten people, and it's more common in women than men. The cause is not entirely known, but iron, folic acid, or magnesium deficiency can bring it on. Stretching and yoga postures can be very helpful. Talk to your health care provider if you think RLS is a problem for you.

Pain. There is very good evidence that acupuncture, massage therapy, yoga, meditation, and relaxation practices can reduce pain and a reliance on pain medications. A physiatrist or integrative pain physician can counsel you about a variety of approaches to ease your discomfort.

Medications. A number of medications can cause sleeplessness, including those that are taken for:
- Colds and allergies
- Asthma
- High blood pressure
- Heart disease
- Thyroid disease
- Birth control
- Pain

- Depression (especially selective serotonin reuptake inhibitor [SSRI] antidepressants)

If you're on any medications—prescription, over-the-counter, or dietary supplements—take all of them to your pharmacist and ask if any could be interfering with your sleep. If they are, talk to your prescriber about other options.

Psychiatric or neurological disorders. Depression, anxiety, panic disorders, dementia, Parkinson's disease, and others can disrupt sleep patterns. Try any or all of the strategies outlined in this section to improve your sleep, and explore therapies such as cognitive behavioral therapy, psychotherapy, and other mind-body approaches that help people cope with stressors in life.

Hormonal fluctuations. Roughly 40 percent of women transitioning through menopause complain of sleep disruption, and many women have trouble sleeping around menstruation. Herbs such as chasteberry are particularly good for menstrual-related insomnia, while black cohosh, hops, and schizandra can be useful for menopausal women.

Disruptions to the sleep-wake cycle. Shift work and traveling across time zones are two of the big culprits for this. Melatonin supplements can help with jet lag when traveling east, but not as much when heading west. On the day of departure, take 1 to 3 mg of melatonin at 6 to 7 p.m. home time and then take it at the local bedtime the first three to four days after arrival. There is less evidence that it's helpful for shift workers.

R℞ PRESCRIPTION FROM DR. LOW DOG

Staying Asleep

The following tips will help you stay asleep:

- If you have a digital bedside clock or clock radio with blue lights, trade it in for one with red digits or an old-fashioned alarm clock.
- Make your bedroom pitch-black, removing anything that illuminates your room while sleeping. Use blackout curtains if necessary.
- Turn down your thermostat to between 60 and 65°F at night.
- Use dimmed night-lights in hallways and bathrooms, and avoid turning on bright lights when getting up during the night.
- Eliminate all caffeine after lunchtime, and limit alcohol consumption to no more than one serving a day.
- Do vigorous exercise early in the day; it increases stress hormones, making you feel more awake. Evening exercise should be nothing more strenuous than walking and stretching.
- Spend at least 20 to 30 minutes outdoors in natural sunlight every day to reinforce the body's circadian rhythm.
- If you live where there is noise at night, put on some white noise, sounds of nature, or soft music to put you to sleep.
- Melatonin signals the body that it's dark outside and time to prepare for sleep. Studies show that taking 1 to 3 mg of

melatonin 45 minutes before your desired bedtime can be particularly helpful for those who have a hard time falling asleep and for jet lag, especially when traveling east. Consider taking an herbal blend containing valerian, hops, California poppy, and/or lemon balm if you have trouble staying asleep. These herbs have long been used as mild, non–habit-forming bedtime remedies.

Illness

⌒

Healing may not so much be about getting better, as about letting go of everything that isn't you—all of the expectations, all of the beliefs—and becoming who you are.
—RACHEL NAOMI REMEN, M.D.

Although no one likes getting sick, it happens to us all. Just like being born and dying, it's a part of life. As a physician, I can tell you without hesitation that the best way to cope with illness is to stay as healthy as possible. We want to be able to mount a strong defense, whether fighting off a cold or a cancer. It's important to recognize that even in the midst of illness, your body is trying to return to its natural state of health. Fever is designed to mobilize the immune system to deal with infection. Diarrhea helps rid the body of bacteria, viruses, or parasites in the intestinal tract. Fainting helps cope with a lack of blood in the brain by forcing the body into a horizontal position that allows blood and oxygen to flow more easily to the brain. The body is designed to be self-healing, and the many ways it maintains equilibrium are nothing short of miraculous.

With few exceptions, such as inherited genetic disorders, the vast amount of sickness we experience occurs when the homeostatic, or balancing, mechanisms of the body become overwhelmed. This can be the result of many things. Eating

R̲X̲ PRESCRIPTION FROM DR. LOW DOG
Simple Tools to Cope With Illness

- Learn as much about your condition as you can so that you can make wise decisions regarding treatment. Be proactive in your care.

- Find a health care provider who is willing to take the time to listen to your questions and concerns, believes that healing is always possible, and is knowledgeable about your illness.

- Consider building a "team" of practitioners. A dietitian, massage therapist, or acupuncturist might have unique insights that can help improve your sense of well-being.

- Whenever possible, choose the least invasive and least risky treatment that is still effective. Sometimes changes in diet, supplements, and exercise can be as beneficial as pharmaceuticals, and with no side effects.

- Involve supportive and nonjudgmental family and friends. Explain how important it is for you to take your medication at regularly scheduled times or why you're changing your diet.

- Be on the lookout for depression. Chronic disease can increase your risk for dark moods. Read up on the symptoms of depression, and let your health care provider know if you're heading in that direction.

- Consider participating in a support group for those with your condition rather than journeying through treatment alone. You can do this in person or online—the important part is to reach out. Isolation isn't good for your mental or physical health.

■ Believe in your heart that you can be healed, even when cure is not possible. Do not let your illness define you.

■ Continue to have outside interests. Ask others about their day. Make time to be in nature. Read inspirational quotes or books when times are difficult. Take slow, deep breaths.

■ Find one thing to be grateful for every day.

---

a diet heavy in high-glycemic-load carbohydrates (processed foods, white bread, white potatoes, candy, and so on) can overwhelm the body's ability to maintain healthy blood sugar. Too much stress and salt can overwhelm its ability to maintain normal blood pressure. Too much alcohol impairs the liver's capacity to function properly. Not getting enough sleep and proper nutrition can weaken the immune response and result in a greater risk of infection. Emotional turmoil can result in depression. In other words, we lose our resiliency when our life is not in balance.

Because we get sick for different reasons, we must treat the body, mind, emotions, and spirit as an interconnected whole. This is the foundation of integrative medicine. When a woman comes to my office for her first visit, I spend an hour listening to her story and asking questions that allow me to understand who she is. It's just as important to know about her friends, family, dreams, faith, beliefs, diet, exercise habits, and sleep patterns as it is to know about her high blood pressure, depression, and fatigue, because all these things are intertwined.

I also tell my patients to remember that getting sick is something we experience—it's not who we are. Although it's a part of us, it doesn't define us. One of the lessons that illness teaches, if we are willing to listen, is that balance and harmony are the keys to health and the paths to healing—balance in our approach to life and harmony in our relationships with the world around us. Healthy food, physical activity, and managing stress are fundamental to our physical health; nature, beauty, art, literature, and music can help heal our mind; and relationships, faith, contentment, and gratitude can provide sustenance to our spirit. When our life is in balance, we experience well-being, even in the face of disease.

Carl Jung said, "He who looks outside, dreams; who looks inside, awakens." I believe that getting sick often forces us to look inward, and if we allow it, illness can help us awaken to our true self.

When I was diagnosed with cancer in 2009, my mind wrestled with all the "why me? why now? why this?" questions. I'd always eaten a healthy diet, watched my weight, didn't smoke, and exercised regularly—all the things you're supposed to do to stay well. But I'd also maintained an unhealthy workload for decades. Although very happy with my work and career, I'd worked 60 to 70 hours every week for years on end. I never used all my vacation days, forfeiting weeks at the end of every year. I was healthy, so I seldom took a sick day.

Looking back, I realize that I wanted to be everything to everyone all the time: a great mother, great wife, great physician, great daughter, great friend, great supervisor, great teacher, great speaker—not good, not OK, but great. I was strong, smart, and hardworking. I'd been told I could have it all. And I could, we can—but at a price. Do I believe I caused my cancer? No. Do I think my workload affected my health? Yes. When I learned I had cancer, I knew things had to change or I'd be dealing with another illness in the future, perhaps one much harder to treat.

Being sick shifted the way I looked at my life, my work, and my family. It made me prioritize what was important. Whether I lived for one more year or another 50, how would I want to spend that time? I'd always made my children a priority, followed closely by my career. Because of this, I'd chosen to live in a town where my kids could easily see friends and I could avoid a long commute to work.

But I'd always dreamed of living in a log cabin in the mountains of northern New Mexico or Wyoming, a place where I could ride my horses and walk through the forest. The dream hadn't wavered in 30 years. It just never seemed to be the right time. That is, until I got sick. Then, as often happens when we give voice to our dreams, the most amazing property appeared. My husband, Jim, and I found a 185-acre ranch nestled into towering Ponderosa pines and Douglas firs in the mountains of New Mexico. It had an old log cabin, barn, and pasture for horses. And the forest felt so alive—mule deer, elk, black bears, foxes, coyotes, rabbits, squirrels, hawks, grosbeaks, robins. I knew I was home.

I've often thought it ironic that if I hadn't gotten sick, I wouldn't have found the home of my heart. I'd still be working an insane amount of hours, trying to be what I thought everyone wanted or needed me to be. I wouldn't be writing this book.

No one wants to get sick. I didn't want to get sick. But illness ended up being one of my greatest teachers. It taught me to pay close attention to my life and not put off my dreams until some future date, for that future is at best uncertain. Modern medicine cured my cancer, but it wasn't until I let go of all the expectations and beliefs that no longer served me and stepped fully into the life that was mine that I felt healed. Martin Luther King, Jr., said, "Only in the darkness can you see the stars." Sometimes, it takes a tragedy for us to awaken and go in search of our dreams.

I always ask my patients these questions: If you knew you had only one year to live, what would you do differently? How would you prioritize your life, your relationships, and your work? Would you take time to make memories that will be cherished long after you're gone? Have you told the people in your life how much they mean to you and how your life is richer because of them? Would you slow down to allow space for the small stuff—a Saturday afternoon picnic, a game of cards with friends, baking cookies with your kids, taking a long bath with music and candles, or enjoying a date night with someone special?

One of the greatest lessons that illness teaches is to not put off what's important, to live life fully. Even when we can't be cured of our disease, healing is always possible. I've been at the bedside of those who died more healed than many who lived very long, healthy lives. Healing is about being whole. It's about letting go of the illusion of who we are supposed to be and making peace with who we are.

Part III

AWAKENING THE SENSES

I go to nature to be soothed and healed,
and to have my senses put in order.
—JOHN BURROUGHS

WHEN I SAT DOWN to write this section of the book, I decided to take a few brief minutes first to walk around my living room, with the intention of opening my senses and observing the fullness of my life. It's winter as I look out the window, and I see in the moonlight that the forest is pregnant with snow, the ground twinkling with crystals, the heavy boughs of the pine and Douglas fir bending down in homage to the earth. I look down at the stream that sings me to sleep all summer. It's quiet now, frozen like glass.

I travel back through time, as I look up at the stars in the night sky, knowing their brilliant light has been traveling hundreds, thousands, even millions of years to reach me. Some no longer exist, having burned out long ago. I turn and see the flames in our stone fireplace burning blue and orange, the mesquite and pine logs crackling and popping. I notice that the heat makes me feel deeply relaxed, almost sleepy. The river stones of the hearth are smooth to my touch, worn down over the millennia by wind and water. The cats and dogs are sleeping on the floor, soaking in the warmth of fire and family. The soft melodies of an acoustic guitar coming from the stereo sound familiar and soothing.

I pick up my glass of red wine, noticing the delicacy of the glass, and then inhale the sensual aroma and savor the taste of berries and oak on my tongue. My eyes look over at my husband and lover, who's sitting by the fire reading, glasses perched low on his nose and wearing faded blue jeans and a black long-sleeved T-shirt. His face is richly tanned from working outside on the ranch. He looks slender and strong, his graying hair the only hint of his aging. I smell a faint aroma of musky spice, and I realize he's wearing the cologne I bought him for Christmas.

I marvel at the number of impressions my senses have processed in such a short time. I notice that I feel calm and centered, filled with gratitude for this brief snapshot of my life. I make a mental note to do this exercise again.

The brain's capacity to take in, process, and store the sensory information of our lives dwarfs the capacity of the world's most sophisticated computer. The dynamic interplay of our senses and our mind allows us to internalize our experience of the external world. What we perceive through our senses influences how we think, how we feel, and ultimately, how we live.

The refinement of our senses is the result of millennia of evolutionary pressure. Our ancestors' survival depended on their ability to discern edible from poisonous plants, distinguish sounds and smells of prey and predator, detect movement in the environment, recognize the tracks of different animals, find water, and much more. Humans huddled together in the open savanna of Africa were vulnerable to the elements, starvation, injury, and attacks by wild animals. The ability to hear and smell an approaching lion could spell the difference between life and death. Our ancestors' senses allowed them to respond quickly to danger through a rapid fight-or-flight response. Now, though, this rapid reaction to sensory input, although still necessary for survival, can have deleterious effects on our health because the level of sensory stimulation is so great.

Sensory overload happens when the sensory experiences from our environment are too much for our nervous system to process and manage. Our bodies perceive this as highly stressful, and our primitive alarm system is activated. We can overload our senses simply by trying to do too many things at once. Driving a car while watching out for other cars on the road, talking to friends, texting, thinking about where we're going, hearing the radio blaring as we speed along at 50 miles an hour—all pretty intense for senses that evolved at pedestrian speeds!

At home, we help the kids with homework while preparing dinner, checking email, and listening to the news anchor talk about the dangers of terrorism and how the country is on the brink of recession. Our nervous system wasn't built for this level of sensory stimulation. It can handle it for brief periods, but when it's ongoing, we end up in a state of perpetual tension, our bodies reacting as if they're on high alert all the time.

Although overload is one problem, deprivation is another. We deprive our senses of many things that nourish and soothe them. Not getting enough quiet time and solitude leaves us feeling wound up and out of sorts. As I discuss in the sections on gardens and nature, research shows that walking in a garden or in nature reduces stress, lowers blood pressure, and shuts down the fight-or-flight response. Listening to soothing music, doing meditation, reading poetry, or using positive imagery can decrease pain, ease anxiety, and improve mood. Using essential oils like bergamot, orange, or lavender can increase our ability to focus, ease depression, and relax. Taking time to slow down before a meal allows us to smell and appreciate the taste of our food and sets the stage for healthy digestion. In other words, it's important to expose our senses to beauty and the delicate, softer sides of our world.

Much of my work in integrative medicine is directed at helping people maintain healthy mental, physical, social, and spiritual connections. These connections are highly dependent on our five senses. Information about our world comes through these sensory channels, which feed directly to our brain. Our sensory experiences are then woven into the fabric of what we call experience, memory, and imagination. Through our senses, we fully experience the richness of our world—the faces of friends and family, the taste a delicious meal, the sound of a running stream, the smell of the desert after a summer rain, or the kiss of a lover. Through the senses, we feel compassion for pain and suffering. All of these impressions linger in our mind and within the recesses of our soul. They are, in essence, what make us who we are.

Touch

*. . . a heart that never hardens, and a temper
that never tires, and a touch that never hurts.*
—Charles Dickens

When I was a girl attending Sunday school,
I heard the story of Jesus and the leper.
The teacher told us that lepers were people with leprosy, a terrible skin disease
that ate away the flesh and was believed to be highly contagious. Lepers were outcasts and unclean; no one would touch
them, not even their families. The Gospel of Mark tells of
a leper who fell on his knees and begged Jesus to cure him.
In his deep compassion, Jesus reached out and touched the
leper, and the leper was healed. I was deeply moved by that
story. Even as a child I'd learned that there were people who
weren't wanted, who went unseen and untouched. That story
was in part what motivated me to study massage, so that I
could learn how to use my hands to heal.

One morning in 1989, I was racing to my office in Las Cruces, New Mexico, trying not to be late for my first massage
appointment of the day. When I arrived, one of my employees
asked to speak with me privately. She told me that the client I was about to see had AIDS and what appeared to be
bruises and sores all over his arms. She asked me to cancel the

appointment. I entered the massage room, where the lights were dimmed and a very thin man in his mid-30s lay on my massage table under a flannel sheet.

Having overheard our conversation, he told me in a weary voice that I didn't have to massage him if I didn't want to. When I saw the bruises on his arms, my heart softened. As I massaged him, tenderly, he began to weep. He didn't cry; he wept. I put my hand over his heart as he said, "I'm sorry, it's been so long since I've been touched. I'm dying and I feel so all alone."

He told me about his partner/husband who'd died a few months earlier, and all the friends he'd loved who'd lost their fight with this wretched virus. I ached for him. The story from childhood played in my head and I thought, these are the lepers of my time—reviled, feared, and even hated. I felt his incredible loneliness and silently prayed, "Lord, let me be an instrument of thy peace." I imagined my hands were filled with light and compassion, and for a time, there was just the two of us. I never saw him again. He died just a few weeks after our visit. This was a chance encounter, two spirits traveling this earthly realm, connected only through touch.

Physical touch is so powerful. It allows us to communicate a wide range of emotions: anger and violence, or comfort and compassion. Touch is the primary way we experience our world as babies. Through rocking, caressing, and holding, babies learn to associate touch and warmth with safety and love. These early experiences are crucial for our ability to form deep attachments later in life.

Touch is so critical that its absence can drastically impair the healthy development of an infant's body and brain.

When Mary Carlson, a professor at Harvard, visited an over-crowded Romanian orphanage, she found rows of babies lying neglected in their cribs. There weren't enough workers to care for all the children, so they were rarely touched even when being fed. Many of the infants were below the third percentile in weight and height, some showing profound failure to thrive. It's thought that lack of touch causes metabolism to slow, lowering the need for nourishment. This metabolic slowing would be a critical survival tool if a young animal were somehow separated from its mother. Taking in less nourishment and dedicating fewer internal resources to growth would increase its chance of surviving until it was reconnected with its mother.

Tiffany Field, director of the University of Miami's Touch Research Institute, found that when premature infants were massaged for 15 minutes three times a day, they gained weight 47 percent faster than those left alone in their incubators. Not only did the babies gain weight, but they were also more active and responsive, suggesting that their nervous systems were also maturing at a faster pace.

The beneficial effects persisted. Eight months after discharge, the babies who'd been massaged scored better on mental and motor ability than those who weren't touched. Dr. Field's decades of research have shown that massage benefits all babies, as well as older children and pregnant women. It can relieve their lower back pain, and lessen tension, stress, and depression after the baby is born. I'm a strong believer in infant massage, and I regularly massaged both of my children.

Teaching someone to administer a very basic massage doesn't take much time or money. Dr. Field trained elder volunteers to do infant massage and then had them massage infants and toddlers in a nursery school setting for four weeks. She also arranged for the volunteers to receive regular massages for four weeks. At the end of the study, researchers found that the volunteers had fewer doctor visits, less anxiety, fewer symptoms of depressed mood, and better sleep. Interestingly, the most improvement was seen when volunteers were *giving* massage. What a beautiful way to bring more touch into the lives of children and improve the lives of our elders!

Healers, shamans, priests, and midwives have always known the gift that lies within our hands. More than 2,000 years ago, the Greek physician Hippocrates declared, "The physician must be experienced in many things, but assuredly also in rubbing." Medicine has gradually transitioned from high-touch to high-tech, and as a result, physicians don't receive training in massage, and many find it of little therapeutic value. Older nurses have told me that many years ago, they'd give hospitalized patients a back rub to help them sleep. Now, as one said, "We just give 'em sleeping pills." Trust me, most patients would prefer a massage to a pill.

But the tide may be turning. An increasing number of hospitals are starting to offer the services of licensed massage therapists. California's Stanford Hospital has been a leader in the field, offering massage for patients both in and out of the hospital for more than 15 years. This makes good sense from both a medical and quality-of-life perspective, as research shows that massage reduces both anxiety and pain. According to Swedish researchers, this is because massage activates the same part of the brain as opiates, explaining its soothing, analgesic effect.

PRESCRIPTION FROM DR. LOW DOG

R℞ Keeping in Touch

- ■ We all love the feel of soft, warm fabrics against our skin. Wrap up in a soft, cozy blanket in the evening and enjoy a cup of tea.

- ■ Get a massage. Don't consider it a luxury; think of it as part of your health plan. For a licensed massage therapist in your area, visit the website of the American Massage Therapists Association at *www.amtamassage.org.*

- ■ Give yourself a massage. You can use many simple techniques to get rid of headaches, neck pain, and tight muscles. A great book is *Healing Self-Massage* by Kristine Kaoverii Weber.

- ■ If you have a child or grandchild, ask your local hospital or massage school where you can take a class to learn how to give infant massage. According to Dr. Tiffany Field, babies like slow, firm, gentle strokes.

- ■ Take a bath. Water soothes, comforts, and relaxes. Enhance the experience by adding some essential oils (see suggestions in the section on smell).

- ■ Hug your pet. Animals are wonderful companions. When you're feeling lonely or down, petting a dog or cat can be a great de-stressor.

- ■ Kiss someone. Few things are more wonderful than the feel of a lover's lips or your lips pressed gently upon the face of a child.

Humans have intuitively understood the powerful connection that exists between touch and consciousness. One of the dramatic ways this is revealed is in the number of metaphors we use that link the two. Think of how our experience with texture and weight influence our language. We all know what's meant when someone says, "I had a *rough* day," "The meeting went *smoothly,*" "*Hold* on to that thought," or "It *weighed* heavy on my mind."

The ability to gauge temperature is another important aspect of our sense of touch. Humans, indeed all mammals, are deeply drawn to warmth. The warmth of our mother's womb and the warmth we felt snuggled next to her body filled us with feelings of safety and security, which later translated into our feelings about other people and situations. We are attracted to someone with a *warm* personality, and avoid those who are emotionally *cold*. It is indeed our sensory experiences that allow us to comprehend metaphoric language.

Researchers at Emory University scanned the brains of volunteers as they listened to textural metaphors and their literal counterparts: "He is wet behind the ears" versus "He is naive," or "It was a hairy situation" versus "It was a precarious situation." The language-processing parts of the brain were active when hearing all of the phrases. However, sentences that included textural metaphors also activated the parietal operculum, a region of the brain involved in feeling different textures through touch. Our brains are literally calling on our experience with physical touch, remembering when we felt something rough, to comprehend the metaphor.

We are all born with a need for healthy, appropriate touch—touch that heals and comforts and never hurts or harms, like the joy that comes from holding hands, from giving and receiving a hug or kiss, from the gentle hand on our shoulder that tells us everything will be OK. It's not surprising that even though our senses of sight, hearing, taste, and smell will eventually diminish with age, our sense of touch never fades. For all that science uncovers about the healing effects of touch, there's so much that's impossible to measure. How do you measure the way touch nourishes our spirit or brings comfort to the sick or dying? Our need to be touched is as basic as our need for oxygen. Without either, we perish.

I'd like to close with a story of the power of touch that my son, Mekoce, gave me when he was five years old. I'd been working an insane amount of hours and had come down with a really bad gastrointestinal infection. My friend Ellen, who was a nurse, had come by to bring soup and check on us when I suddenly had a seizure. I was on the floor, not conscious of my surroundings, when Mekoce knelt on the floor beside me, put his small hands over my heart, and closed his eyes. Ellen asked him to move so she could check on me, but Mekoce said, "No, I have to stay here and take care of my mom. I have magic in my hands."

He closed his eyes again and sat very still. A few minutes later, when I started to rouse, Mekoce gave Ellen a big smile and told her the magic had worked!

Ellen had tears in her eyes when she told me the story several hours later. I gently took the hand of the young soul sleeping next to me and allowed the healing gift of his love and faith to flow through me. I sometimes imagine a world where we all believe we have magic in our hands, the kind of magic that has the power to convey our deepest love and, without any words at all, to say, "I know it's dark and you're scared, but I'm here; you're not alone."

Sight

The eye is the window of the human body through which it feels its way and enjoys the beauty of the world.
—LEONARDO DA VINCI

We humans are highly visual creatures. Sight is central to our experience and dramatically impacts our well-being. We devote more of our brain to vision than to any other sense, because sight requires coordinating our environment, our eyes, and our brain. How we see, both physically and emotionally, affects our lives and our health.

In the purest sense, the world is revealed to us by light. It's the energy by which we see. In dim light, we can only discern shapes in black and white. In full light, we see a world rich in form, color, and texture. When wavelengths of light strike an object, they are either absorbed or reflected. The light that is reflected enters our eye. Muscles in the iris, the beautifully colored part of the eye, expand or contract to control the amount of light that enters the pupil, opening more when it's dark, less when it's bright.

Light travels through the pupil until it reaches the lens, a transparent, flexible structure that fine-tunes the image before projecting it onto the retina. Here, the light is mapped as an image by the activation of a series of light-sensitive cells known as rods and cones. These specialized cells convert the light image into electrical impulses that are transmitted via the optic nerve to the visual cortex in the brain. The brain then creates a three-dimensional impression of what the image is and where it is, giving it meaning and form. Multiple parts of the brain must work together at lightning speed to keep up with the vast number of images being taken in by our eyes. And it all happens without any conscious thought on our part.

Because vision is such a highly complex process, there are a number of areas where trouble can occur. Let's consider the lens. When I turned 45, I reluctantly bought my first pair of reading glasses. This was to be expected, because as we age, our lenses stiffen, making it harder to see things up close, a condition called presbyopia. People who are farsighted, or have hyperopia, also cannot focus on things up close, but in this case, the lens isn't the problem. The eyeball is either too short or the cornea, the clear membrane covering the eye, has too little curvature, so light entering the eye is distorted. The opposite is true if you're nearsighted, or have myopia. You can see close objects clearly, but objects farther away look blurry. This occurs if the eyeball is too long or the cornea has too much curvature.

Cataracts are another problem that can affect our lens. They form when the lens is damaged by too much exposure to ultraviolet (UV) light. As the lens becomes cloudy, objects look blurry and out of focus. Cataracts can be surgically corrected, but the best approach is to prevent them by wearing sunglasses that filter out 100 percent of UV light. A 2010 review in *Ophthalmic Research* also concluded that supplements of lutein and zeaxanthin—the pigments that protect plants from excessive UV light—help prevent cataracts.

Although the lens, cornea, and shape of the eye are important for vision, the major player is the retina. If it's damaged,
we're very likely to lose some or all of our vision. Age-related
macular degeneration (AMD) is the leading cause of vision
loss in Americans over 65. The macula sits right in the center
of the retina and is responsible for the sharp, central vision
needed for reading, driving, and seeing fine detail. In some
people, as the cells and blood vessels in the macula age, they
begin to thin and degenerate. As more of the light-sensitive
cells in the macula break down, vision slowly gets worse.

The Age-Related Eye Disease Study (AREDS), sponsored by
the U.S. National Institutes of Health's National Eye Institute,
found that taking high levels of antioxidants and zinc reduced
the risk of developing AMD by about 25 percent. Fish oil,
lutein, and zeaxanthin are also being studied in AREDS-2, as

PRESCRIPTION FROM DR. LOW DOG
Warding Off Eye Problems

In the Age-Related Eye Disease Study (AREDS), the following
vitamins were found beneficial:

- Vitamin C: 500 mg
- Vitamin E: 400 IU
- Beta-carotene: 15 mg (25,000 IU)
- Zinc (as zinc oxide): 80 mg
- Copper (as cupric oxide): 2 mg

Talk to your health care provider prior to using these.

newer evidence suggests they slow the progression of AMD. If you've been diagnosed with AMD, talk to your eye doctor about these supplements and about the implications of diet in general. According to a study from the University of Sydney, diets with a high glycemic load also increase the risk for AMD (see the section on food for more information on glycemic load). And if you smoke, stop!! Smoking damages the blood vessels in your eyes, increasing your risk for AMD and accelerating its progression.

Another major threat to the eyes is diabetes, because it's hard on the nerves and blood vessels, including those in our eyes. One of the leading causes of blindness in American adults is diabetic retinopathy, caused by abnormal changes in the blood vessels that lead to fluid leakage, swelling, or bleeding in the retina. Diabetics also have double the occurrence of glaucoma, another leading cause of blindness in the United States. Given all this, it's important to reduce the risk of diabetes by getting regular physical exercise and ditching foods that increase insulin resistance.

A healthy diet and lifestyle can protect our precious gift of sight, and as sure as the foods we eat affect our health, so do the images we digest. Every day, our eyes send hundreds of thousands of bits of information to the brain, where the information is processed, encoded, packaged, and stored. I can close my eyes and see the faces of my newborn children. Feelings of intense love well up inside me. I can also remember the image of my Grandma Jo in her coffin, still and lifeless. Visual memories are among our strongest. We can pull up experiences and impressions from times long past. And it's happening mostly without our conscious thought.

Think about that for a moment. Our eyes, and our minds, are taking in endless amounts of images, and we give very little thought to how they might be affecting us. In 1972, the U.S. Surgeon General warned that viewing violent images on television could be unhealthy for children. Television rating systems were put in place, though surveys show the vast majority of parents don't use them. In 2011, the Supreme Court overturned a California ban on the sale of violent video games to minors, citing First Amendment protection and lack of clear evidence that they cause real harm.

Let's be clear: There *is* evidence that violent media, especially for children, can have adverse effects on health. A 2009 policy statement from the American Academy of Pediatrics read, "Research has associated exposure to media violence with a variety of physical and mental health problems for children and adolescents, including aggressive behavior, desensitization to violence, fear, depression, nightmares, and sleep disturbances. More than 3,500 research studies have examined the association between media violence and violent behavior; all but 18 have shown a positive relationship." They went on to note that the strength and quality of the evidence is stronger than that for tobacco use and lung cancer, calcium and bone mass, condoms and HIV prevention, and lead exposure and low IQ.

I don't believe everyone who watches violent media or plays violent video games turns into a rapist or murderer. I know it's more complex than that. But as a parent, I didn't allow my kids to play violent video games or go to violent movies. Even without evidence of harm, I'd still find these media morally objectionable and counter to the teachings of

R𝑥   PRESCRIPTION FROM DR. LOW DOG
For Eye Health

- If you have dry eyes, wear contact lens, or have had Lasik surgery, consider taking a fish oil supplement that provides 1,000 mg EPA and 500 mg DHA a day. A study from the University of Texas Southwestern Medical Center found that when patients with dry-eye syndrome were given omega-3 fatty acids, tear production and volume dramatically increased. By the end of the study, 70 percent of those in the omega-3 group were asymptomatic, compared with only 37 percent of those taking the placebo.

- To help prevent cataracts, wear sunglasses with 100 percent UV protection. A daily dose of 10 mg of lutein and 2 mg zeaxanthin may also decrease the risk of cataracts and AMD. Talk to your eye doctor about taking these supplements if you have or are at high risk for AMD.

- Use natural lighting as much as possible. When using artificial light, choose full-spectrum LED bulbs when doing focused work such as reading or sewing, and consider full-spectrum fluorescent bulbs when looking for a light that is evenly distributed over a larger area. Fluorescent bulbs should be covered to prevent eyestrain or headache.

- Wear safety goggles or a face shield when you're working with hazardous chemicals or anything that might break and send small particles into your eyes.

- When doing focused work, whether reading a book or working on a computer, take a five- to ten-minute break every hour and use artificial tears if needed to reduce eye irritation.

compassion that I wished to instill in my children and cultivate in my own heart.

Media, like art, can also have positive, beneficial effects on mood and behavior. A 2010 review in the *Journal of Pediatrics* found that child- and teenage-directed media could help build antiviolent attitudes—empathy, tolerance toward people of other races and ethnicities, and respect for elders. *Sesame Street* is a prime example of this kind of television, but shows like *Friends* and *Grey's Anatomy* have also been shown to convey positive educational messages to teenagers. As far as video games go, parents can encourage neutral games like *Tetris,* or pro-social games like *Super Mario Sunshine, Lemmings,* or *Chibi-Robo!* for young gamers. A multinational study led by Douglas Gentile from Iowa State University found that pro-social games actually increased helping behaviors, cooperation, sharing, and empathy in adolescent and university undergraduate gamers in Singapore, Japan, and the United States. Life is about choices. When possible, choose beauty and joy.

Create beauty in your home by making spaces where you can gaze on forms and colors that soothe and inspire. Photos of family, colorful candles, statues, plants, and flowers are all soft to the eyes. Find a window that has a nice view. Put a chair where you can sit and look outside, watching nature change as you travel through the seasons. Enjoy television and other media but do so consciously, with thought for what you're viewing. Our eyes, beyond their wondrous gift of sight, are also metaphors for life. When we lose sight of our purpose, we struggle to perceive that which can only be seen with the heart. As Marcel Proust wrote, "The real voyage of discovery consists not in seeking new landscapes, but in having new eyes."

Eye Screening Schedule, Recommended by the American Optometric Association

Patient Age	Examination Interval	
	Asymptomatic/ Risk-free	At Risk
Birth to 24 months	At 6 months of age	At 6 months of age or as recommended
2 to 5 years	At 3 years of age	At 3 years of age or as recommended
6 to 18 years	Before first grade and every two years thereafter	Annually or as recommended
18 to 60 years	Every two years	Every one to two years or as recommended
61 and older	Annually	Annually or as recommended

Nature

Everybody needs beauty as well as bread,
places to play in and pray in, where nature may heal
and give strength to body and soul alike.
—JOHN MUIR

Some of my fondest childhood memories were of times spent outdoors. I would sell Girl Scout cookies every year to help earn the money my troop needed to go to summer camp. Two glorious weeks of sleeping in big green military-style tents, cooking meals over a campfire, singing songs, staying up late at night telling ghost stories, and learning how to identify animal tracks and steer a canoe. I wore my mosquito bites with pride and regaled my parents with endless stories of my adventures.

My grandparents had a lot to do with my love of nature. They owned a sportsman's supply store near Dodge City, Kansas, filled with fishing rods and reels, sleeping bags, cook stoves, tents, and everything else needed for a successful camping trip. At the ripe old age of six, I learned to bait a hook and caught my first catfish sitting on a dock at Clark County Lake with my Grandma Jo. She was strong and beautiful, knew how to fish, shoot a rifle, set up camp, and, with her eighth-grade education, how to manage the account books for her store. When we were out camping and fishing, she would tell me the stories of her childhood and what it meant to be part Comanche. From her, I developed my love of storytelling.

Like most children, I loved to play outside with the neighborhood kids. When I came home from school, Mom would say, "Take off your school clothes, then go outside and play. Be home for dinner." She would never tell us to go do homework. That was for after dinner. We were to go outside and play and "burn off all that energy." I can tell you, it was a long afternoon for mothers and kids on the days when it rained, and we had to play board games inside.

Outside, we were free, and our imaginations were as big as, well, as big as we could imagine. There was never a stick that couldn't become a sword or a magic wand, or a rope swing on a tree that couldn't be transformed into a jungle vine complete with Tarzan, Jane, and Cheetah. We played tag, hide-and-seek, and hopscotch. We caught horned toads and lizards, and let them go. We were a part of nature and nature was a part of us—there was never any sense of being "disconnected."

I believe that for us to be whole human beings, we must be mindful of this deep and intimate relationship with nature. In an attempt to explain this need to be close to nature, Edward O. Wilson, the Harvard naturalist and Pulitzer Prize winner, coined the term *biophilia*, which literally means love of life or love of living things. Wilson postulates that we are drawn to nature because we evolved in natural spaces filled with trees, grasslands, flowers, and water. It is in our genes, so to speak.

Science has shown that the human brain prefers to look at images of landscapes and green spaces rather than images of concrete, glass, and steel. When we see natural spaces, the parahippocampal cortex, a part of the brain rich in endorphins, is activated. Endorphins are chemicals in the brain that help reduce pain, relieve stress, and give the immune system a boost. Thus, when we look out at a beautiful landscape, we experience pleasure, our blood pressure goes down, our heart rate slows, our muscles relax, and our immune system is better able to fight off infection.

This has broad implications for our health. In 1984, Roger Ulrich published the results of a groundbreaking study in *Science* that found when patients recovering from surgery were able to look out their window at a view of trees and nature, they had significantly shorter hospital stays, took less pain medication, and had fewer complaints than did patients who looked out at a brick wall. Increasingly, hospitals are seeking ways to weave green spaces into their architecture.

When I was recovering from surgery at Tucson Medical Center, my bed looked out into a courtyard with a great big mesquite tree. At one point, a red-tailed hawk sat on a branch for about five minutes, much to my delight. I was up and walking just a few hours after surgery, needed very little pain medication, and went home almost a day earlier than planned. Although no one likes having surgery or being in the hospital, I had nothing but gratitude for my room, my surgeon, and the staff, and I believe that my view of nature had a great deal to do with my attitude.

Could nature also hold the key, at least in part, for children who are living with attention deficit/hyperactive disorder (ADHD)? Richard Louv, the author of *Last Child in the Woods*, thinks it just might. He uses the phrase *nature-deficit disorder* to describe the increasing separation children have from natural spaces when they grow up in urban areas and/ or spend a lot of time indoors watching television or playing video games. He also talks about the potential consequences of that separation.

In his book, Louv cites a number of studies showing the positive benefits of green space on the behavior and attention of children with ADHD. This is confirmed by other research that finds when schoolyards include green space and when environment-based education is integrated into the curriculum, improvements in test scores for reading, math, science, and social studies result, as well as a reduction in discipline problems in the classroom.

A majority of Americans and other people around the globe live in urban environments, and I don't think this will dramatically change in the near future. I frequently travel to big cities for meetings and speaking engagements, but I live in the middle of a forest in northern New Mexico. Most of my time is spent with my senses "wide open" so that I can take in everything around me: the fragrant smell of pine and of the forest after a hard rain, the squawking of blue jays, the rustling of the wind as it moves through the trees, the sight of elk and deer as they wander through our meadow, the brilliance of a billion stars on a clear night.

By contrast, when I travel to New York City or Chicago, my senses are completely overwhelmed by the sound of car engines and honking, people rushing and trying to stay out of one another's way, neon signs that light up the night, street vendors trying to sell things, the delicious smell of ethnic cuisine

PRESCRIPTION FROM DR. LOW DOG
Five Ways to Experience Nature

1. National, state, and city parks. These unique places preserve our spaces of nature's beauty and bounty. Here's a website link to find a park near you: *www.nps.gov/find apark/index.htm*.

2. Books on nature. One author that I would highly recommend is Richard Louv. His words from *The Nature Principle* brought tears to my husband's eyes as we listened to him speak about saving our children from "nature-deficit disorder."

3. Your backyard. Wherever you live, you can experience nature by going outside. The amazing thing about nature is that it adapts and is everywhere. You can help by creating an environment where you live.

4. Natural history museums. Explore the history of life on Earth! These museums offer exhibits teaching about life on Earth. Many programs for children and adults inspire wonder, discovery, and responsibility for our natural and cultural worlds.

5. Local botanical gardens. Explore the uniqueness of your local area plants. Botanical garden centers celebrate, cultivate, and conserve the rich botanical heritage and biodiversity of our region. Most areas have clubs to support you in your gardening efforts.

followed a few seconds later by the horrid stench of garbage. Although I love the shopping, the theater, the phenomenal restaurants, all the culture and activity of big cities, I understand why people who live there have higher stress levels: Their senses take in so much information that the brain and nervous system become frazzled. Unlike the sights and sounds of nature, which are hardwired into our genes after millennia of living in nature, the sights and sounds of technology and urban living are foreign and harder for the brain to process.

An interesting study that researchers from the University of Michigan conducted divided people into two groups and had one group walk for 50 minutes in the Ann Arbor arboretum and the other walk for 50 minutes in downtown Ann Arbor. After a week, the groups switched places. Before each of the walks, researchers assessed the mood, memory, and attention of the participants. When the participants returned from their respective walks, the assessments were repeated. Researchers found that when people walked in the arboretum, their attention, memory, and mood all improved. When they walked in the city, they performed worse than before their walk on every test!

Marc Berman, one of the researchers involved in the study, posits that this happens because the brain must be extra vigilant when walking in the city. You have to avoid getting hit by a car, navigate around other pedestrians, and choose to ignore or act upon all the stimuli telling you to eat or shop. Being in the city is hard work for your brain and nervous system, and it takes a toll.

It's important to remember that you can bring nature into your life no matter where you live. In fact, studies repeatedly show that even small forays into natural spaces can be restorative and healing. For those who live in the city, visiting a park where you can take a walk—alone, with a friend, or with your pet—or just sit and drink a cup of tea can have a tremendous impact on your sense of well-being. Do you have trees in your yard? If so, put some comfortable chairs on the porch and sit outside before or after dinner. Are you near a lake, river, or the ocean? Make a point to take the family out a couple of times each month for a picnic or a walk along the beach. Although nature is best when experienced in these ways, researchers tell us that even simple things like putting green plants in your home and workspace or hanging pictures of landscapes on the wall can lower stress levels.

In some cases, maybe the best prescription a physician could write would be for a hike in the mountains, a bike ride along the river, a walk in the garden, or a weekend camping trip. The point is that nature is good for your mental and physical well-being. Bring more of it into your life.

Smell

❦

The smell and taste of things remain poised a long time, like souls, ready to remind us . . .
—MARCEL PROUST

Smell is often overlooked as a minor player in the symphony of our senses, but it is what allows us to delight in the aroma of a favorite food or the fragrance of a perfume or flower. Our sense of smell also acts as a warning system, alerting us to dangers like gas leaks, spoiled food, or fire. With every breath, we inhale our world. Everything we can smell is emitting volatile chemicals that float through the air until reaching the back of our nose. The more volatile, or easy, it is for the molecules to evaporate, the stronger the smell. The reason cooking makes food smell stronger is because heat increases the volatility of aromatic molecules. Of course, some things can't be smelled: Stones, steel, and glass are nonvolatile solids. On average, humans are able to distinguish approximately 10,000 different smells, but because of genetic differences, no two people smell exactly the same aroma.

The volatile aromatic molecules move up through our nostrils until they reach the back of our nose. Then they float upward until they become trapped in the mucus covering millions of odor-receptor cells, or olfactory neurons, which catch

PRESCRIPTION FROM DR. LOW DOG
Making Essential Oil Blends

Certain blends can help or heal various states. Just mix equal parts of the oils listed on each line and you'll have the therapeutic aroma you need:

- Passion: jasmine, rose, and clary sage
- Meditation: myrrh, frankincense, and juniper
- Menopause: clary sage, frankincense, and geranium
- PMS: clary sage, lavender, and cypress
- Colds: thyme, eucalyptus, and pine
- Tension: bergamot, clary sage, and frankincense
- Depressed mood: rose, sandalwood, and neroli
- Loss and grief: rose, marjoram, and cypress
- For the bath: Put eight to ten drops in a tub of water and soak.
- In a vaporizer: Put five to eight drops in an aromatherapy vaporizer and let it run in the room you're in.
- For a massage: Put five drops in 1 tbs of almond, apricot kernel, or safflower oil.
- Skin spritzer: Put eight drops in a 2-oz bottle of water with a pump sprayer. Mist yourself as desired.

and identify the scent molecules. The other way aromatic molecules arrive at this location is through a channel that connects the roof of the throat to the back of the nose. When we chew our food, odor molecules are released and travel through this opening until they reach the odor receptors in our nose. If this channel is blocked, for instance by a cold, odors cannot reach the olfactory neurons, and we're unable to appreciate the flavor of our food. No matter the pathway it takes, once the aromatic molecule binds to the olfactory neuron, a signal is sent along your olfactory nerve to the smell center in the brain, located within the limbic system.

The limbic system contains the amygdala, which houses both our emotional memory and olfactory center. That's why aroma and emotional memory are intricately linked. Using brain-imaging techniques, researchers have shown that when we inhale an aroma, the amygdala is activated. The stronger the emotional response to the smell, the more the amygdala lights up. Smells can be associated with a particular person or an experience with which the odor was repeatedly paired.

For instance, rose water always conjures up memories of my Grandma Jo, and Old Spice makes me think of Grandpa Glenn. Many times, though, we're not aware of any specific memory; we just have a positive or negative association with a smell and don't know why.

Research is now showing that our emotional associations with certain smells may start in the womb. A baby can readily recognize the smell of its mother, even without seeing her. Studies have shown that during periods of separation, if a newborn is able to smell the odor of its mother's amniotic fluid, it is soothed and stops crying. A study published in *Neuroscience Research* found that babies exposed to the odor of their mother's breast milk had significantly less crying, grimacing, and lower salivary cortisol levels (a stress hormone) when having their blood drawn, compared with babies exposed to odors from other women's milk or formula. The thought that my smell, my very essence, is imprinted into the deepest recesses of my children's memories is pretty cool!

Pheromones are technically chemicals an animal produces that can change the behavior of another animal of the same species. Sex pheromones are extremely powerful attractants for mating. Animals in threatening situations emit alarm pheromones to warn other members of the species of danger. Researchers are busy studying the impact of pheromones on human behavior. Mothers can pick out clothing worn by their children, whereas fathers cannot, but men can readily tell if a T-shirt was worn by a man or a woman.

It may be pheromones that cause women who live or work closely together to menstruate at the same time. George Preti of the Monell Chemical Senses Center in Philadelphia found that after three months of periodically applying the sweat of other women under the noses of female study participants, the participants began to menstruate in synchronicity with the women whose sweat they'd smelled. Julie Mennella, another researcher at Monell, found that smelling the sweat of breast-feeding women increases breast milk production in other nursing women. Who knew there was so much going on with our sense of smell?

Aromatherapy is the art of using aromatic plants for medicine and health. For thousands of years, humans have burned herbs and plants for their fragrant smell, often as part of worship or ritual. The resin from the frankincense tree, considered more valuable than gold, was burned in temples from Egypt to China, and the smoke was believed to carry prayers to heaven. Native American peoples also burned, or smudged, herbs to prepare the mind and heart for ceremony. Today, at prayer lodge, or sweat lodge, ceremonies, bundles of sage and cedar, braids of sweetgrass, and pinches of tobacco are used to purify those taking part, bless the stones in the center of the lodge, and carry prayers to heaven.

PRESCRIPTION FROM DR. LOW DOG
Enhancing Your Sense of Smell

- Because our olfactory neurons tire easily, smell for 2 to 3 seconds, pause for 20 seconds, and inhale again.
- Challenge yourself to find words that describe the aroma. It's not as easy as you think! Wine-tasting books can be great resources, as they have many descriptors most of us wouldn't think of.
- To improve your smell, go for a quick walk. Our sense of smell is better after exercise.
- Eat foods high in zinc like oysters, roasted pumpkin seeds, dark chocolate, and peanuts.
- Humidify the air or purchase over-the-counter moisturizing nasal sprays. Moisture can improve your sense of smell by unblocking your olfactory neurons.
- Make a spritzer and spray it in your room, office, car, or on your pillow for a great way to set the mood.
- Put three to four drops of your essential oil blend on a cotton ball or tissue and put it in your purse, linen drawer, or backpack. It's great for those smelly gym bags too!

Modern aromatherapy uses primarily pure essential (volatile) oils that have been extracted from a plant through a variety of extraction techniques. The result is a small amount of oil that is highly fragrant and that perfumists, flavor chemists, and aromatherapists seek. The global flavor and fragrance industry, much of it based on essential oils, exceeds 20 billion U.S. dollars annually. Although aromatherapy is a small fraction of the industry, it's gaining in popularity, in part because more scientific studies are showing its beneficial effects. Rachel Herz, an expert in smell and a professor at Brown University, reviewed 18 aromatherapy studies and found convincing evidence that odors can affect mood, physiology, and behavior. I use aromatherapy both professionally and personally to reduce body tension, ease stress, and lift the mood.

It's important to protect our sense of smell. Like any of our senses, it can affect our overall health when we lose it. Anosmia, which literally means smell blindness, is the complete loss of smell. Because 80 percent of taste is smell, people with anosmia often experience a loss of appetite and pleasure in eating. A study from the University of Sydney, Australia, found that people over the age of 60 with hyposmia, a reduced ability to smell, had a much greater incidence of depression and poorer quality of life than age-matched control participants with an intact sense of smell. As we get older, the number of olfactory neurons steadily decreases, but some age-related conditions, including diabetes and thyroid abnormalities, can accelerate the process. In disorders that affect the central nervous system, such as Parkinson's and Alzheimer's, the loss of smell is often the first symptom.

Tobacco smoke impairs the ability to identify different odors, so if you want to preserve your sense of smell, don't smoke or let anyone smoke around you. Exposure to certain solvents and chemicals, as well as taking certain medications, can also impair the sense of smell. Although zinc deficiency can make you lose your sense of smell and taste, over-the-counter zinc nasal sprays were linked to more than 130 cases of anosmia. If you feel you're having problems with your ability to taste or smell, make sure you talk to your health care provider or schedule an appointment with an ear, nose, and throat doctor.

Garden

*My garden of flowers is also my garden of thoughts
and dreams. The thoughts grow as freely as the flowers,
and the dreams are as beautiful.*
—Abram L. Urban

S ummer always brings a special kind of joy to my
heart, as the spring planting ripens into an abundance
of green delights in the garden. Plump tomatoes, tender squash, delicate culinary herbs—everything that
makes its way from our garden into our kitchen seems to taste
a little sweeter, smell a little more fragrant, and look a little
brighter than what I buy at the store.

Gardening is a form of meditation—digging in the soil,
trimming back leaves, watering, and weeding. Every day, the
garden must be tended. On our ranch, which sits at an eleva-
tion of 7,800 feet, the sun is very intense in early summer,
and we go many weeks without rain. Shade screens have to
be erected over the plants and watering done by hand late
in the day to honor the delicate balance between conserv-
ing water and bringing forth our food and medicines. When
the afternoon showers begin in late July, there's little need to
water, and the plants appear to grow an inch every day. It's
as if some magic descends on our garden. There's so much
activity, as the bumblebees, butterflies, and hummingbirds flit

about. The flowers create a tapestry of lilac echinacea, scarlet lobelia, and deep purple pulsatilla, and the aromas shift as I move, from the citrus of lemon balm to the heady scent of mint to the earthy smell of valerian. I get lost in my thoughts as I pull the weeds, prune back the withered leaves, snip the flowers on my catnip and oregano, or eat an heirloom tomato off the vine.

The joy of having a garden is something anyone can experience. When my son, Mekoce, was living in Santiago, Chile, doing fieldwork for his Ph.D., he lived in an apartment in the middle of a huge metropolitan area. Mekoce and the young boy in his Chilean host family planted seeds in pots on the balcony. The entire family watched in delight as the seeds grew into beautiful basil and tomato plants for the kitchen. Now back in Berkeley, Mekoce maintains a wondrously rich garden on his apartment balcony and is never short of mixed greens, tomatoes, or fragrant herbs.

Even for those who swear they're too busy or say they don't have a green finger on either hand, creating a garden is so easy. It can be as simple as filling a few pots on the porch with flowers, vegetables, and herbs. Even keeping a few houseplants that you care for can lift the spirits. Whether you have a balcony in the city, a small plot behind your house in the suburbs, or a large space on rural acreage, having a garden can be an amazingly healthy and rewarding experience.

Researchers have found that gardening can reduce stress, lower blood pressure, and boost the immune system. And remember that being outside gives us lots of sunshine and vitamin D, both of which have been shown to improve mood

R℞ PRESCRIPTION FROM DR. LOW DOG
Garden Plants for the Senses

Gardens are a perfect place to engage the senses. Roses are beautiful, lavender smells heavenly, and rosemary is green all year round. These are some of my favorites.

- **Lavender.** The word *lavender* comes from the Latin *lavare*, which means "to wash," a reference to its historic use in bathing. The small purple flowers are highly aromatic and can be added to bathwater or dried and put in linen closets or lingerie drawers.
- **Rosemary.** Rosemary, the herb of remembrance, is a hardy plant for most any garden. Highly fragrant and deep green, it can be used fresh or dried in cooking. Rosemary tea is used as a hair rinse for women with dark hair.
- **Peppermint.** Peppermint, a cross between two types of mint (water mint and spearmint), is a delight to both the nose and the tongue. Peppermint leaf tea can soothe an upset stomach and relieve a tension headache. I love mine iced on a hot summer day.
- **Chamomile.** Known in Spanish as *manzanilla* ("little apple") because of its characteristic smell, chamomile flowers are nature's gift to the stressed and anxious. Very gentle, a cup of tea soothes both young and old.
- **Catnip.** Catnip, a beautiful member of the mint family, is widely known for its effect on cats. But in humans, catnip leaf makes a delightful beverage tea, calming the spirit and quieting the stomach.

- **Lemon balm.** Referred to as the "gladdening herb" during the Middle Ages, this gentle member of the mint family is a premier stress reliever. In fact, German health authorities have approved the use of lemon balm for anxiety and poor sleep brought about by tension and worry.
- **St. John's wort.** St. John's wort is so named because the plant blooms in late June, the time of the feast of St. John the Baptist in Europe. A beautiful plant for the garden, this herb is one of the best studied for minor depression.
- **Basil.** Basil, a staple of Mediterranean foods, should be a staple in any culinary garden. Fresh basil is far superior to dried. Just puree with olive oil, garlic, pine nuts, and Romano cheese for a delicious pesto.
- **Oregano.** Oregano is another popular herb in Mediterranean cooking. But like most culinary herbs, it is excellent for relieving colds and nasal congestion and settling an upset stomach. I pinch off a small leaf whenever I stroll by, just savoring the aroma.

---

and overall health. Surveys repeatedly indicate that when people spend time in a garden, whether a public space or their own, they report a positive change in mood, less tension, and an easier time thinking and coping. People with dementia who are in treatment facilities that incorporate gardens have less aggression, anxiety, and agitation than those in facilities without gardens. This means less medication and lower stress for residents, their families, and the staff. Imagine what our world would be like if we spent more of our money investing in gardens of flowers and herbs and less on antipsychotics and tranquilizers.

In addition to the pure joy that being in a garden brings, the garden itself is in many ways a metaphor for life: The growing cycle has a rhythm that teaches us about birth, abundance, maturation, death, and rebirth. This metaphor has meant different things to me at different stages of my life. To start with, there is the preparation of the soil so seeds will grow. Like many women, I had a strong connection to this aspect of gardening when I was pregnant. I wanted to eat healthy, get extra sleep, and manage my stress so that the "soil" would be optimal for the child growing within me.

At other times, I have envisioned my body as a garden in which I strive to tend the soil and plant the seeds of health. I think this metaphor for tending the body is even more pronounced for those of us who have dealt with cancer or suffered a heart attack. And then there is the pruning and weeding, a never ending job in the garden and in our lives. Getting rid of the withered leaves and clearing out weeds is essential for ensuring healthy plants. There have been many, many moments in my life when it was time to take a good look at what I was carrying around and weed out whatever no longer served a purpose—from activities to habits and negative thoughts that kept me from fully taking in the richness of my life.

Harvesting what has been sown is especially satisfying to gardeners. Watching the plants bring forth their gifts is nothing short of miraculous. I still marvel at how the lowly tomato plant in May becomes a gentle giant held within its tower by late August, its fruit ripe and luscious. Though this miracle happens every summer, I still feel like an awestruck child when I watch my garden come to life. It also causes me to reflect on the years when I was too busy to prepare the soil adequately, not thoughtful about what I planted, or lazy when it came to pruning and weeding. Those years I had little to harvest.

When I moved to Tucson, Arizona, for example, I thought I could simply grow the same plants I had when I was living in northern New Mexico. I couldn't. The heat was so intense and the climate so dry that much of what I planted the first year didn't survive. When I talked to experts at a local plant nursery, they gave me tips on plants I could grow that wouldn't use lots of water and could tolerate the heat. My garden thrived the next year. As I watched it come to life, I wondered how many times in my life I had tried to plant something in an environment that wasn't conducive to growth.

In many ways, I believe women are like a garden. We each come with our own soil, climate, and internal environment. Some seeds we plant will never grow; others will grow with exceedingly hard work every day. But when we plant seeds that are well suited for our environment and our nature, they grow with just a modest amount of work.

Taste

⌒

Live each season as it passes; breathe the air,
drink the drink, taste the fruit, and resign
yourself to the influences of each.
—HENRY DAVID THOREAU

When I sat down to write this section, I thought it would be a good idea to grab a few things from the kitchen to put me in the right mood. As I eat a piece of 72 percent cacao bar with hazelnuts, I take in a hint of bitterness, a crunch of nut, and the glorious aroma of chocolate. I pinch my nose and take another nibble. Even though I know that 80 to 90 percent of taste is through smell, I'm still surprised at how bland the chocolate now tastes.

I sit for a few minutes organizing my thoughts and then bite into a small sliver of lemon. My mouth puckers at its sour taste, and I smile as I enjoy it. That exquisite yellow color, intense citrus aroma, and burst of sour: Lemons always make me feel happy.

Next is a Pink Lady apple. It looks perfect, and I eat two slices, thinking about how sweet and moist it is. I understand why apples have always been one of my favorite fruits. I move on to the pretzel, crunchy and salty. Even this small amount of salt feels a little overwhelming, and I realize that I'm not a

Enhancing Smell and Taste

- Spice up your meals! Even if your senses of taste and smell aren't working well, the nonspecialized irritant nerve cells are still highly operational. These are what make you cry when chopping an onion or what makes your nose run when you eat hot chili peppers.

- Have a picnic in the mountains. Many people believe that food tastes better when they're camping. The reason for this is that at higher altitudes, the lower air pressure causes volatile molecules to vaporize more quickly, which improves both their smell and taste.

- Reset your taste button. Eliminate all sugar and salt for one week. I know that doesn't sound like it would be fun, or easy, but if you do it, you'll find that everything tastes so much sweeter and saltier. It's amazing. This is the best way to control your sweet tooth or cut back on salt.

- Take a tour of your plate. Take bites of the different foods on your plate to prevent your olfactory nerves from getting bored. The more aromatic your food smells, the better it tastes.

- Avoid really hot food and drink. We've all burned our mouths and damaged our taste buds. The good news is that our taste buds are constantly being replaced about every seven to ten days.

- Stay hydrated. As we chew our food, it mixes with saliva, which enables food molecules to bind to our taste receptors. A dry mouth decreases taste.

big salt fan. Finally, I cut a sliver of hard Parmesan cheese and let it soften in my mouth. Then, with my eyes closed, I slowly chew it. Oh, it's so delicious and the taste so unique.

When I was growing I up, I learned in school that there are four basic tastes: sweet, sour, salty, and bitter. This had been accepted as fact since the time of Aristotle, more than 2,000 years ago. But, in fact, there are at least five tastes. In 1908, Kikunae Ikeda, a chemist at Tokyo Imperial University, set out to discover what accounted for the unique taste he found when eating asparagus, cheese, and meat, tastes clearly different from sweet, sour, bitter, and salty. Working in his lab, Ikeda found the ingredient was glutamate (glutamic acid), one of the most common amino acids in nature. We now know that there are specific glutamate receptors on the tongue. The amino acid must be freed from its protein matrix through aging, drying, roasting, fermentation, toasting, or ripening to produce glutamate's distinctive taste, which in honor of Ikeda, is called *umami*, "delicious flavor," in Japanese.

Taste is what makes eating such a pleasurable experience, but it was also critically important to the survival of our early ancestors. They needed to distinguish edible plants from poisonous ones, many of which are extremely bitter. It should come as no surprise then that our taste preferences, including an intense dislike for bitter, begin while we are still in the womb. Ultrasounds show that after the 14th week of pregnancy, the baby is able to control the swallowing of amniotic fluid; when alcohol or nicotine are present in the mother's blood, the baby swallows less, presumably because it doesn't like the taste. From the 16th week on, the baby shows a clear preference for sweet-tasting substances. When such substances are injected into the amniotic fluid, the infant sucks and swallows more. When bitter is introduced, the baby closes its mouth to prevent swallowing.

It is to our evolutionary advantage that young children are so averse to bitter. Babies put everything in their mouths. Learning not to swallow bitter-tasting foods even before birth offers some protection against swallowing poisonous plants. But babies are more sensitive to taste than adults, in general, as they are born with taste buds on the tongue and the sides and roof of their mouth, intensifying taste. As we grow older, the taste buds disappear from everywhere except our tongue, making us less sensitive to taste but able to enjoy a broader range of flavors such as bitter greens, coffee, alcohol, and spicy foods, as they aren't perceived as intense. Scientists have confirmed what parents have always known—little kids can be picky eaters, so pick your battles carefully when it comes to mealtimes. Don't fight over food.

Our mouths contain roughly 10,000 taste buds, most of which are located in the tiny bumps—papillae—on the tongue. Each of these taste buds contains between 50 to 100 specialized taste receptors, and each of these projects a tiny taste hair that detects food molecules dissolved in our saliva. This is one of the reasons our mothers always told us to chew our food slowly! The longer food lingers in the mouth, the more time it has to mix with saliva and interact with the taste buds.

Each taste hair is specially designed to respond to one of our five tastes. Contrary to popular belief, there are not separate areas of the tongue that distinguish among tastes; we can taste everything everywhere on the tongue. When the tiny hairs on our taste receptors are stimulated, nerve impulses are sent to the brain's limbic system and the frontal cortex. The limbic system explains why we may have strong emotional feelings associated with certain tastes, while the frontal cortex identifies the taste and makes sense of the emotional experience.

When my son, Mekoce, was two years old, we went out to dinner with my parents. The adults were busy talking and didn't notice that Mekoce had eaten about half the butter that had been set out for bread. A few hours later, no surprise, he vomited. For years, he was unable to eat anything with butter on it. That was his limbic system at work. As he grew older, he realized that eating small amounts of butter wouldn't make him sick, and he starting using it on toast or in cooking. This is because his frontal cortex, the thinking part of his brain, was able to override the emotional memory connected to eating butter.

Taste isn't experienced in isolation; smell and sight also play a role. Many people who think they've lost their sense of taste have actually lost their ability to smell. When you have a bad cold, the aroma molecules can't waft up through the throat to the olfactory bulb or reach the back of your nose, so food tastes bland. You can lose your sense of smell and taste if the nerves in your head are damaged from an accident, from a disease like Parkinson's, or from radiation treatments for head and neck cancer. If the nerves are damaged, the impulses from the tongue or nose can't reach the brain for interpretation. Neurologists and ear, nose, and throat doctors are specialists who evaluate loss of taste (and smell).

The way food appears is also important, and all great chefs know that presentation is almost as important as taste and smell. It's not just thinking a worm might *taste* bad that makes us not want to eat it; it's *seeing* wiggly worms on our plate that would do most of us in. But associating taste with appearance is generally a learning process, as a study published in the *Journal of Food Science* found: When people were given cherry drink colored greenish-yellow, 40 percent thought it tasted like lemon-lime, not cherry! Our brain gets confused when food looks like one thing but tastes like something else. When I was five years old, my brother handed me what he said was cola. Being thirsty, I took a big drink. It was room-temperature coffee! My brain was expecting something sweet and got something bitter. To this day, I've never taken another drink of coffee.

We can do many things to awaken our sense of taste. I truly believe that by slowing down to enjoy and appreciate the flavors of our food, we will eat less, have fewer digestive troubles, and bring back the pleasure of mealtime.

Hearing

True silence is the rest of the mind; it is to the spirit
what sleep is to the body, nourishment and refreshment.
—WILLIAM PENN

Whenever I think about our sense of hearing, the song "Good Vibrations" by the Beach Boys starts playing in my head. That's because what light is to sight, vibration is to hearing. Sound is a vibration or series of vibrations set in motion by an object. Vibrations create sound waves that travel through space until they reach our ears and strike our eardrums, causing them to vibrate at roughly the same frequency as the original source. Sometimes that resonance can be very powerful.

I remember the first time I heard a Tibetan singing bowl, used for meditation and prayer in Asia for centuries. I was in a meditation class, and my teacher took out a bronze bowl and began to move a leather-wrapped stick slowly around the rim. The bowl produced the most incredible deep ringing. I could feel the sound vibrating inside me, as if it was coming from within me. Total resonance. She stopped after a couple of minutes, and we began to meditate. It was one of the most powerful meditation practices I'd ever experienced. Tibetan singing bowls have been used for meditation and prayer in Asia for centuries.

Vibrations are transmitted from the eardrum into the middle ear, where they are amplified before heading into the fluid-filled, labyrinth-like structure called the cochlea in the inner ear. The cochlea contains 15,000 to 20,000 specialized sensory cells with tiny hairlike projections, called cilia, which pick up the tiniest vibrations in the cochlear fluid. If the cilia are destroyed by loud sounds, they never grow back, and permanent hearing loss results.

The sensory cells convert the vibrations into nerve impulses that are sent via the acoustic nerve to the sound-processing part of the brain, the auditory cortex. Many parts of the brain work together to interpret the sounds we hear, particularly musical sounds. Because music is so complex and can have such a profound effect on our emotions, I've dedicated an entire section to the topic.

For thousands of years, the sounds being processed in our brains were those of nature. Birds chirping, the wind moving through the trees, the humming of bees, and the utterances of other people—these sounds resonate in the ancientness of our minds. Loud music, airplanes, horns honking, trains, sirens, heavy machinery, televisions blaring—these are relatively new vibrations in the evolutionary orchestra. And they can take their toll on our health. The Environmental Protection Agency tells us that noise pollution adversely affects the lives of millions of people and that it can add to stress-related illnesses, high blood pressure, hearing loss, sleep disruption, and lost productivity.

The decibel (dB) scale is used to measure the loudness of sound. Zero dB is the quietest sound most people can hear, though there are some individuals that can hear minus 5 or even minus 10 dB. The maximum time you can safely expose your hearing to 85 dB is 8 hours; however, that time shrinks to just 15 minutes for sounds 100 dB or higher. With the iPod and MP3 player revolution, there is growing concern about the impact of listening to music at high volumes through earphones for hours at a time. According to the American Academy of Audiology, noise-induced hearing loss affects about one out of every eight children in the United States. I shudder to think what I did to my hearing standing up at the front of those concerts I went to in my youth!

Noise-induced hearing loss can increase the risk of developing tinnitus, a ringing or buzzing sound heard when the brain isn't processing other sounds. From the Latin *tinnire,* which means to ring, tinnitus affects 12 percent of men and 14 percent of women in the United States over the age of 65. There are

R℞ PRESCRIPTION FROM DR. LOW DOG
Know Your Decibel Levels

Normal conversation	60 to 65 dB
Busy street	75 to 85 dB
Lawn mower/heavy traffic	85 dB
Hand drill	98 dB
Motorbike	100 dB
Nightclub/car horn	110 dB
Music player on loud	112 dB
Chain saw	115 to 120 dB
Rock concert/ambulance siren	120 dB

potentially hundreds of causes of tinnitus, hearing loss being one of the most common. Certain drugs are ototoxic, meaning that they can cause hearing loss either by damaging the cilia in the cochlea or weakening the messages sent from the acoustic nerve to the auditory cortex. Aspirin and many over-the-counter analgesic medications, including ibuprofen and naproxen, are well known for causing ringing in the ears, but this is usually reversible when you stop taking them. Certain antibiotics and cancer drugs can also cause tinnitus, and some antidepressants make tinnitus worse if you already have it. Sometimes you can experience spontaneous tinnitus when in complete silence, as the brain tries to orient itself to the absence of ambient sound.

Tinnitus can be difficult to treat. An evaluation by an ear, nose, and throat doctor, usually followed by a referral to an audiologist, is an important first step. Many people get tremendous benefit from using a Neuromonics device, which is approved by the FDA for treating tinnitus. It works by transmitting white noise through headphones specifically programmed to mask tinnitus. By generating sound, the spontaneous activity and hyperactivity in the auditory cortex is lowered and tinnitus is dramatically reduced. Other sound generators that can be worn on the ear to produce white noise and provide relief are also available.

While decibels measure the loudness of sounds, frequency measures the range of sounds we can hear. Frequency is measured in cycles per second, called hertz (Hz). Humans are able to hear sounds with frequencies ranging from 20 Hz to 20 kHz (20,000 hertz). We can hear higher frequencies when we're young, but as we age, the eardrum stiffens and our ability to hear high-pitched sounds declines. Frequencies higher than 20 kHz (ultrasounds) and lower than 20 Hz (infrasounds) are inaudible to the human ear. Many animals, like dogs, cats, and bats, can hear sounds in the ultrasound range, and dolphins hear up to 150 kHz, more than seven times higher than us mere mortals.

The ability of bats and dolphins to echolocate—find objects by reflected sound—has been adapted and incorporated into modern medicine. Ultrasound machines use high-frequency sound waves to visualize structures inside the body. When the sound waves bounce back, the "echo" is captured, and the image is recorded for viewing by the radiologist. Through ultrasound, many women see the image of their unborn baby for the first time. Ultrasound is also used to help heal sprains by sending vibrations into the tissue, reducing inflammation and pain by bringing better blood flow into the area. Sonar uses sound waves to detect other ships, determine ocean depth, and even locate schools of fish.

Less known are infrasounds, a topic I became interested in after watching a PBS show that included an interview with a Thai survivor of the tsunami that devastated Southeast Asia in 2004. The man told the reporter that minutes before the tidal wave landed, his elephants became highly agitated and stampeded up a nearby hill. He believed they *sensed* the tsunami was approaching. Countless other stories are told of animals acting very strangely minutes before a catastrophic natural event. Scientists know that earthquakes produce distinct infrasound pulses that can travel thousands of miles at speeds far faster than a storm surge, in the case of a typhoon. It's highly likely that some animals, like whales and elephants, are able to hear and react to these sounds.

PRESCRIPTION FROM DR. LOW DOG
For Better Hearing

The following tips will help you protect your hearing:

- If you can't avoid being in a very loud environment, wear hearing protection. Look for products with noise-reduction ratings (NRR) of 22 dB or greater. You can find them at most pharmacies and drugstores; most concert venues sell them, too, so you can rock to the music while preserving your hearing.
- Wear "active" noise-canceling headphones when listening to music. These headphones emit sound waves that cancel background noise, allowing you to keep the volume down. Noise-canceling earphones are not as effective because they typically use "passive" canceling techniques (think earplug).
- If you need to raise your voice to be heard over the television or music, it's too loud. Turn down the volume.
- If you have tinnitus, talk to your health care provider about a hearing assessment. Make sure you tell your doctor what medications you're taking. For great unbiased information, go to the website of the American Tinnitus Association (*www.ata.org*).
- Eat a low-glycemic-load, Mediterranean-style diet. If you don't eat fish, take an omega-3 fish oil supplement. A multivitamin that provides the recommended daily intake of beta-carotene and vitamins E and C will give added protection.

■ Cigarette smoking and breathing secondhand smoke is bad for your hearing (and health overall)—one more reason to quit smoking and to not allow others to smoke in your house, car, or office.

Though we can't hear these sounds, some of us might be able to "sense" them. British scientists Richard Lord and Richard Wiseman played four pieces of live music in a London concert hall filled with 750 participants who were asked to describe their reactions while listening to the music. The audience didn't know that some of the music had been laced with infrasound, but one in five listeners reported feeling uneasy, getting chills down the spine, feeling sad, or experiencing fear when it was present in the music.

It must have been incredibly disconcerting to "sense" these low-frequency vibrations without being able to hear them consciously. But it's likely part of our evolutionary biology. Earthquakes, volcanoes, storms—these are all big and terrifying events; over the millennia, we've come to associate these low-frequency sounds with things that are dangerous. And scientists believe that infrasound is what lies beneath many of our fears and apprehensions attributed to the phenomenon of ghosts and haunted houses. How so? Do we "sense" an infrasound and attribute it to a spirit?

Vibrations influence and affect our lives in many ways. The ability to hear sound is central to acquiring speech and understanding language. Children with hearing problems that go unnoticed and/or untreated often do poorly in school and suffer from lower self-esteem. People with hearing loss, especially young people, experience greater social isolation, making access to hearing tests and hearing aids critically important. A study in *Ear and Hearing*, the journal of the American Auditory Society, found that with each increment of hearing loss, there was a 5 percent increase in depression and 7 percent increase in loneliness among 1,511 people under age 70 who'd taken a national hearing test. An Italian study found that when hearing aids were provided for individuals over age 70 suffering from both hearing loss and depression, there was a dramatic reduction in depressive symptoms and significant improvement in quality of life for both the participants and their caregivers.

Adopting a healthy lifestyle based on exercise, a low-glycemic diet (see the section on food, pages 49-74, for more on this), and no exposure to tobacco smoke is fundamental to preserving our hearing. Chemicals in cigarette smoke can damage the cilia in the inner ear and restrict blood flow to the middle and inner ear. Diet and exercise can help prevent diabetes, which causes nerve damage in the cochlea, impairing transmission of auditory signals to the brain. A study in *Diabetes Care*, the journal of the American Diabetes Association, reported that the odds for developing low- to mid-frequency hearing impairment are 100 percent in diabetics. Researchers at the University of Sydney in Australia found that people with the highest intake of foods high in glycemic load had a 76 percent greater risk of developing hearing loss. Eating a low-glycemic, Mediterranean-style diet will also ensure plenty of beta-carotene, vitamin C, and omega-3 fatty acids, which have also been shown to help prevent noise-induced and age-related hearing loss.

I've relied heavily on my hearing all my life. Because my dyslexia made speaking and reading so difficult, I learned to listen. It took forever to read a page and even longer to write one, but I could remember in exquisite detail every word the teacher said. I not only remembered the words but every inflection or nuance in her voice.

The ability to listen has served me well as a physician. In *How Doctors Think,* Dr. Jerome Groopman tells us that on average, physicians interrupt their patients within 18 seconds of the start of their conversation. Because of the way medicine is structured today, many physicians feel driven to get information in a quick, efficient manner and arrive at a diagnosis and treatment plan within a 15-minute appointment. But a lot of important information is missed in such a short process. A diagnosis is important, but only within the context of the individual's life. To understand that, doctors have to listen to a patient's story. The more I am able to *listen* to a person's story, the better I'm able to truly *see* them and help them on their journey toward health.

In all our encounters, it's important to listen generously, to lean in and hear what is being said, even in the pauses between the words, and to speak softly in response. An ancient proverb says that a gentle answer turns away wrath, but a harsh word stirs up anger. Spend a day paying attention to the sounds of your world. What music is playing? How loud is it? What is the vibrational tone of your home? Is it buzzing with laughter, brimming with anger and yelling, singing with joy? Are you a good listener, allowing others to finish before jumping in? Do loud noises intrude upon your solace? Many people grow so accustomed to the noise and chatter of their lives that they no longer really listen.

Find ways to reawaken your sense of hearing. Bring more soft and natural sounds into your life. Play CDs of nature while working. Use white noise or sounds of nature when going to sleep or to dull the noise of traffic or neighbors. The sound of birds, ocean waves, raindrops, and wind are familiar and comforting to the brain. Make time for quiet; allow your mind to rest. Embrace silence. For only in the quiet do we hear the voice of our own heart, sometimes the sweetest sound of all.

Music

Music cleanses the understanding; inspires it,
and lifts it into a realm, which it would not reach
if it were left to itself.
—HENRY WARD BEECHER

My mother used to joke that I was born with a phonograph needle in my mouth! That's because I was always singing. I inherited the gift of song from my Grandma Jo, who had a beautiful alto voice. She and I would ride in the back of a pickup truck or sit around a campfire singing every verse we knew to "She'll Be Coming Round the Mountain," "Camptown Races," and "Pass the Biscuits, Mirandy." As I grew older, I learned to play the guitar, and was deeply drawn to the late 1960s and '70s folk music of my generation. I need music. I use it to energize me when cleaning the house or working out on the elliptical. I keep a variety of CDs in my car so I can listen to whatever I'm in the mood for. I love the singing of birds when I'm out in the garden. I start and end my day listening to soft jazz. For me, a day without music is like a day without sunshine.

We each have a personal experience with music. It has a unique way of conveying our deepest emotions and moods. It is the language of our feelings. From the haunting sitar and beauty of classical Indian music to the spellbinding sounds of the didgeridoo in the Aboriginal music of Australia, peoples from around the world and across the span of time have been moved by the power of music. Although modern music is largely secular and relates to our day-to-day experience, music has its roots deep in spirituality and religion. Hindu philosophy is interwoven with the harmonies of India, Buddhism influenced the music of Asia, and music continues to play a major role in Christian worship and Jewish prayer services.

As a child, I remember going to intertribal powwows and becoming lost in the sounds of high-pitched voices and the steady beating of the drum. The repetition of the verses and the power of the percussion carried me to a place of heightened spiritual awareness, a place beyond ordinary reality. The transcendent quality of music brings many of us into a deeper state of worship and prayer. If poetry is the language of the heart, music is the language that speaks to our soul.

Music's physiological effects on us are incredibly complex. Unlike the spoken language, music integrates auditory, memory, and learning-related structures in an extremely elaborate fashion. The whole process starts with a vibratory source that initiates the sound. The source could be our vocal cords, clapping hands, the strings on a guitar, or the movement of air through a wooden or metal instrument. These vibrations strike our eardrums and are converted into nerve impulses that travel through the temporal lobes and limbic system, stimulating pathways associated with language and memory and releasing neurochemicals that affect our mood. Listening to music is like weaving the threads of our psychological selves with the threads of our physical selves into a brilliant multicolored tapestry.

Studies have shown that softer, simpler melodies relax and soothe, while complex harmonies arouse. One Italian research team monitored breathing, blood pressure, heart rate, and cerebral blood flow in 12 experienced singers and 12 people with no musical training as they all listened to six different

R℞ PRESCRIPTION FROM DR. LOW DOG
Tieraona's iPod Playlists

Add to your life by creating musical playlists to live by. Here are six of mine:

1. T's Memory Songs: Having been a music lover ever since I can remember, I created this list to remember the times of my life and the music to go with it.

2. Songs to Work By: This is a selection of instrumentals that allow me to concentrate.

3. Kitchen Music: A lively group of my favorite songs, this is the playlist that gets my daughter, mother, and me in the mood to dance while cooking.

4. Soothe: Music has the ability to create your mood. After a long day, it's a treat to play this list and have a glass of my favorite wine with my husband.

5. T's Dance Mix: This is similar to the Kitchen Music playlist, but I'm not cooking!

6. T's Commuter Songs: I have a 90-minute drive to the airport (which I visit too frequently), and this list makes the time fly.

musical styles. The study, published in *Circulation*, the journal of the American Heart Association, found that slow or meditative music induced relaxation, while faster tempos increased focused attention, blood pressure, heart rate, and breathing. But what was interesting was that after listening to any form of music, all participants were more relaxed than before. Singing has similar effects on our physiology, reducing stress, improving oxygenation in our blood, encouraging deep breathing, and focusing the mind.

Neuroplasticity is the ability of the brain to adapt to change and experience, and music definitely enhances this ability. Learning music can actually change the structure and function of the left temporal lobe, the part of the brain responsible for the mental processing of speech. A study in *Neuropsychology* found that musical training in children significantly increased verbal memory—the ability to recall and comprehend words. Learning songs or how to play a musical instrument is very similar to memorizing poems or long pieces of prose, which also enhances memory and recall. Charles Emery, a researcher at Ohio State University, found that patients who exercised while listening to music—in this case, the *Four Seasons* by Vivaldi—had almost double the ability to remember lists of words (verbal recall) compared with those who exercised without music.

The impact music has on the brain opens up many possibilities for helping those who are neurologically impaired. Although we don't fully understand why people who've lost their ability to speak can often sing, or those who've lost their memory can recall songs, we do know that music can help the brain heal. A Finnish study found that verbal memory and focused attention improved significantly faster and better in stroke patients who listened to the music of their choice for two to three hours each day for two months as opposed to patients who listened to audio books or nothing at all.

Normally, after having a stroke, patients spend the first few weeks in their rooms with limited interaction. Listening to music during this critical time period could enhance cognitive recovery and prevent depression. Similar findings on memory and cognition have been documented in studies of healthy elders and those with mild forms of Alzheimer's dementia. Physicians have encouraged "mental exercises" like doing crossword puzzles or learning a foreign language to preserve memory and keep the mind sharp, and science now shows that listening to music can have similar effects.

Some of the effects we see from music may be due to the fact that it can trigger the release of dopamine. This neurotransmitter, or brain chemical, is associated with happiness, reward, arousal, motivation, and pleasure. (Drugs of abuse, like cocaine and methamphetamines, increase the release of dopamine, which is why they can be so addictive.) When researchers at McGill University used functional magnetic resonance imaging (fMRI) to monitor the brain changes of study participants listening to music, they found that the intense pleasure experienced in response to music is due to the release of dopamine from nerve cells in the nucleus accumbens.

And reviewers from the nonprofit Cochrane Collaboration found that music therapy improves mood in people with depression. Most antidepressant medications only work on the other two neurotransmitters involved in mood—serotonin and norepinephrine—and many people who take

Let Music Be Your Medicine

- Listen to music every day.
- Invest in a decent sound system. You will experience the richness of music better if played through a set of speakers rather than through headphones.
- Practice listening to music, not just hearing it in the background but actively listening so that you can distinguish the different instruments, the natural pauses, and the melody.
- Create a variety of playlists for your MP3 player, iPod, or CD player. Make one with lively, upbeat songs you can listen to when exercising, doing work that doesn't require intense concentration, or feeling down. Make another with soft, relaxing instrumental music that can be played when doing focused work, lying down to sleep, or feeling totally stressed out. Create one that has a blend of music, ranging from simple to complex melodies, lyrics that are sad and happy, tempos that are slow and fast, that you can listen to when driving, cooking in the kitchen, and so on.
- Sing along to your favorite songs. Sing as if no one is listening. Sing from your heart.
- Cherish silence. After listening to your favorite music, just sit for a minute or two and experience the silence. This will help your brain integrate all that you have heard.
- If you are interested in working with a qualified music

therapist, or if you are interested in becoming one, visit the American Music Therapy Association at *www.music therapy.org.*

---

antidepressants continue to complain of impaired motivation and loss of pleasure even when their depression improves. These studies suggest that music might offer its own therapeutic benefits in treating depression. I wouldn't hesitate to encourage someone living with depression to talk to a trained music therapist.

Music also increases the production of endorphins, natural opiate-like compounds that reduce our perception of pain. In a study sponsored by the National Institutes of Health, participants suffering from chronic pain were randomized into three groups. The first group selected their own music, the second group picked from preselected tapes of relaxing music, and the third group received no music intervention and served as controls. Participants in the two music groups experienced as much as 21 percent decrease in pain and 25 percent reduction in depressed mood after just one week of listening to music for one hour a day. There was no change in the control group's pain. Reduction in pain relief was similar between the two music groups, suggesting that much of the benefit comes from listening to music we enjoy.

As the research grows, music therapy is being integrated into conventional medicine. More than 30 studies have shown that music reduces anxiety and pain and improves mood and quality of life in people with cancer. Many cancer centers now employ trained music therapists to help patients cope with the stress of the disease and its treatment. Other studies have found that music can reduce anxiety and stress before and during surgery. A German study found that patients who listened to soothing music while undergoing total hip replacement surgery required less sedation and had lower blood levels of the stress hormone cortisol. Less sedation and lower stress means fewer complications and a speedier recovery.

I can vouch for these results, because I don't know how I would have gotten through the hospital stay after my hip replacement without my iPod and headphones. Listening to music cut out the hospital noises and allowed me to go into a deep state of relaxation so that my body could heal. I'm surprised more hospitals don't offer music and headsets to patients. Soft, soothing music playing in the hospital can make patients and their families, as well as medical staff, feel more relaxed.

Although science is revealing the many ways music can be used to improve our health, I admit I'm happy that part of its magic remains a mystery. Music, with its unique ability to speak directly to the heart and soul, is one of our most beautiful forms of expression. It has eased the physical, emotional, and spiritual suffering of countless numbers of humans.

I'd like to finish this section where I started, with my grandmother Jo. She suffered a heart attack at the age of 91 and was taken to a local nursing home, the closest thing to a hospital available in her small town of Ashland, Kansas. Shortly after arriving, Grandma told her dear friend Melanie that she was tired. Melanie said Jo closed her eyes, and with a smile on her face, she began humming a song. And she died. As I sat in the church listening to this story, I felt the immensity of my love and gratitude for all that she'd given me. Not the least was her love of music and the gift of song. From the lullabies we hear as children to the verses of "Amazing Grace" sung at our death, music has the power to comfort, transform, bring unity, and heal. It is my prayer that when my time comes, I too will die with a song on my lips.

Part IV

LISTENING
TO
SPIRIT

Let your mind start a journey through a strange new world. Leave all thoughts of the world you knew before. Let your soul take you where you long to be. Close your eyes, let your spirit start to soar, and you'll live as you've never lived before.
—ERICH FROMM

W E'RE DEEP INTO WINTER on our ranch as I begin to write this final part of the book. After staring at the computer screen waiting for the words to come, I put on my coat and boots and go for a walk in our forest. As my feet carry me softly through the snow, I take in the stillness around me. The beautiful New Mexican sky is a rich blue without a wisp of gray or white clouds. I see the footprints of the coyote and deer that have passed through the field ahead of me. I hear the Steller's jays chattering noisily as I pass by. The snow has a bluish hue and is deep on the northern slopes of our mountain. A hawk soars high above me, wings outstretched, riding the currents without effort.

I begin to sing my medicine song. Mark, a Pueblo man who used to work on the ranch, once told me that the spirits of this land are old and they want you to sing to them. My breath is visible in the cold morning air as my song becomes one with the wind. The Navajo believe *nilch'i*, the holy wind, is what brings life to the people. I close my eyes and inhale my world, remembering the word *inspiration* literally means "breathing in." I walk back to our cabin, content that the words will now find their way to the page.

The word *spirit,* from the Latin *spiritus,* means breath, and from the moment we take our first breath until we take our last, we are imbued with its life force, called by the names *prana, qi,* or *mana* in other languages of the world. All traditional systems of medicine recognize the role of spirit in health and sickness—it is considered a strong ally in the healing process. Yet spirit is given only the smallest nod in modern medical training, which views illness as primarily biological in nature. We identify the pathology or offending agent and then use surgery to cut it out or drugs to destroy or suppress it. Although I'm deeply grateful for the advances science has brought to the field of medicine, there remains much suffering that cannot be alleviated by a scalpel or a pill.

There is a story within every illness and something to be learned from listening to it. Over the years, I've been privileged to hear many stories, each of them as unique as the person who shared it, and yet, woven through them is a common thread: Much of our pain is rooted in our deafness to spirit. We remain in an ongoing struggle to break free from the illusions of who we think we're supposed to be so that we may live the life we are called to live and become the person we were born to be.

Birth is hard for both a mother and child. There are moments when the mother thinks she might die as her body struggles to release the life within. And leaving the warmth and safety of the womb for an unknown world is frightening for a baby.

But the mother must give birth and the child must leave, or they will both die. And so it is with our dreams and our spirit. We must give them life or they will die.

As children, we follow in the footsteps of our parents. But there comes a time when we must find our own way. We'll meet many people along the journey who want to tell us which direction our life should take—some with good intentions, others not. Some whisper that there's only one path, the one they're walking. Follow them or perish. Others say in a loud voice to stay where you are, to stand still, for they've seen the world and it's a dangerous place. Occasionally, we may come across someone who wishes us strength and courage, knowing that there is no path other than the one we're walking and that, to live, we must follow where our individual path leads.

This part of the book is really a collection of thoughts about how to open our hearts and minds to the language of spirit. Children live the language of spirit when they play and use their imaginations. We hear it in joyful laughter. We open to it through forgiveness and when we speak from our hearts. When we nurture our relationships, no matter how few or how small, we begin to create a sacred space for family and community, a place where we can feel safe just being. When we extend that circle of relationships to other creatures, we see that all of life is connected and sacred. Our spiritual senses are opened in solitude, nature, meditation, and prayer. Even though there are tips and ideas scattered within these essays, there is no road map, no ten easy steps to finding your life's purpose.

But when we listen to our spirit, we have the opportunity to fall in love with the essence of who we truly are. We free ourselves from the weight of trying to be everything to everyone all the time. We no longer see ourselves through the eyes of others but through the eyes of the divine. And when we see ourselves in this light, we see the world in the same light.

When we choose to think and act with beauty and compassion, we experience moments of absolute peace and bliss. When we open to life, we see that we all share the same breath, we are of the same spirit, and we are all related. Healing cannot be separated from the world we live in, the food we eat, the air we breathe, the words we speak, or the way we treat others. As we open our heart to spirit, we feel more deeply connected to the world around and within us, and we will sing our medicine song. For in truth, the medicine road that we were set upon when we took our first breath is a spirit road, and if we follow it, we will know what it means to be whole and to be healed.

Humor

⸎

What sunshine is to flowers, smiles are to humanity.
These are but trifles, to be sure; but scattered along life's
pathway, the good they do is inconceivable.
—JOSEPH ADDISON

I remember reading Norman Cousins's book *Anatomy of an Illness* in the early 1980s. It was the story of how he had used humor to heal. In 1964, while editor of the *Saturday Review* and a "citizen diplomat" for the United States, he'd been diagnosed with ankylosing spondylitis, a condition that causes severe inflammation and stiffness in the spine and other joints. After having some adverse reactions to the drugs he was taking, Mr. Cousins decided to take charge of his own health. He asked his doctors to reduce the number of medications he was on and inject him with really large doses of vitamin C. Then he checked himself out of the hospital and into a hotel room where he spent the next few weeks watching Marx Brothers movies and tapes of *Candid Camera,* and reading funny books. He immediately began to feel less pain and to sleep better. Over time, he gradually recovered his freedom of movement and returned to his role as editor.

Many years ago at an herb conference where I was lecturing, I had the pleasure of listening to and sharing dinner with

Dr. Patch Adams, a physician who has spent his career bringing free health care to his community and speaking internationally about the role of humor in health. A fascinating and down-to-earth man, Dr. Adams is also a street clown. He certainly looked the part during his talk at the conference, wearing a clown suit and mismatched socks as he shared his experience of taking 15 clowns to Russia every year to bring humor to hospitals and orphanages.

After traveling all around the world, Patch Adams believes one of the deadliest diseases is loneliness, and the treatments for this—no surprise—are humor and fun, along with love, family, exercise, community, faith, passion, wonder, and curiosity. A movie that bears his name, starring Robin Williams, tells the story of this wonderful man's life and how humor and joy saved his own life as a young college student. I highly recommend watching it.

It seems that both Cousins and Adams were on to something. There is a growing body of evidence looking at the effects of humor and laughter on health. Dr. Lee Berk is a medical researcher at Loma Linda University who has been studying the neuroendocrine and immune effects of positive emotions for many years. His work has shown that laughter can rev up your immune system. In one of his studies, 52 healthy men viewed a humorous one-hour video. Then blood samples were taken, showing that their white blood cells and antibodies were elevated and stayed that way in some cases for up to 12 hours.

One type of white blood cell called a natural killer (NK) cell is particularly increased and activated by laughter. Low NK cell activity is correlated with increased risk of

Prescriptions for More Laughter

- Rent a comedy. Give up the crime show or heavy drama for a night of laughter. Some of my favorite comedies are *Ghostbusters, Airplane!, Monty Python and the Holy Grail, National Lampoon's Vacation, Ferris Bueller's Day Off, A Fish Called Wanda, Finding Nemo,* or any comedy with Jim Carrey.

- Put on music that makes you smile. How about Louis Armstrong's "What a Wonderful World," "Walking on Sunshine" by Katrina and the Waves, "Good Vibrations" by the Beach Boys, or "Love Shack" by the B-52s? Make your own playlist for days when you need an emotional lift.

- Give the gift of laughter. Consider giving a DVD of a funny movie or a joke book to a sick friend. After all, laughter is the best medicine, and it'll last longer than flowers.

- Hang around people who have a good sense of humor. Everyone knows at least one sunny person. Remember, emotions are contagious!

- Pick up a funny novel to read during stressful times. Some books that may tickle your funny bone include *Hitchhiker's Guide to the Galaxy, Bridget Jones's Diary, Lucky Jim,* and *Breakfast of Champions.*

- Never pick up a newspaper without first reading the comics.

- Smile at least ten times every day. Surely you can find ten things to make you smile—birds singing, a child playing, the sun shining, a great cup of tea or coffee. Smiles are the kissing cousins of laughter.

infection and poorer health in people with cancer and HIV. Dr. Berk has also conducted studies that show laughter ameliorates many of the adverse effects of stress by blunting two major stress hormones, adrenaline and cortisol. Numerous researchers have demonstrated the beneficial effects of laughter on the heart as well. For instance, in one study, blood pressure was lowered by 10 to 20 mmHg (points) after a 20-minute laughter session. Other studies have shown that laughter can reduce a person's risk of having another heart attack when used as part of a comprehensive cardiac rehabilitation program.

When Groucho Marx said that a clown is like aspirin, only he works twice as fast, Marx probably didn't know that scientists would one day be able to show that laughter actually increases the body's production of opiate-like compounds called endorphins. The more robust the laughter, the greater the pain relief.

Hospitals and other health care settings are taking this research seriously. A study conducted at the University of California at Los Angeles (UCLA) found that when children watched funny videos, their ability to tolerate pain was increased. Anything we can do to make painful procedures a little easier is a worthwhile undertaking, which is why I'm delighted that many pediatric centers are bringing in clowns to brighten the lives of ill children, their families, and staff. Pain is a complex and debilitating condition requiring a truly integrative approach to its management, but given what we know about the power of laughter, maybe it's time physicians wrote more prescriptions for watching the Three Stooges or cartoons!

There's another type of humor therapy popping up around the country called laughter yoga. Laughter yoga classes combine yogic-style breathing with laughter, and class participants essentially laugh for no reason. No jokes are told, but the instructor leads the class through a series of loud "ho, ho, ho, ha, ha, ha"s. Then participants throw their arms up and heads back and laugh out loud. Instructors next go through a series of laughter exercises.

In the class I was in, we went around shaking hands with each other, making eye contact, and laughing out loud. We were then instructed to act like we were making banana splits and eating them while laughing. The concept behind this is based on evidence that the body doesn't differentiate between fake and real laughter. You get similar physical and psychological benefits from either. I know you're probably thinking this sounds pretty silly, and indeed it is. That's the point. Although I faked my way through the beginning of the class, I was laughing for real by the end.

Having a good sense of humor can also get you through a lot of life's frustrations, as I know well from working with two wonderful women—Moira Andre and Rosalyn dePalo— at the Arizona Center for Integrative Medicine. One of the things the three of us do is plan and execute six one-week conferences for 70 health care professionals every year. No matter how well we plan, things sometimes go wrong and the three of us have to figure out a solution. During our problem-solving sessions, we'll invariably break down in fits of uncontrollable laughter—tears-streaming-down-the-face laughter. That's because Moira has the gift of taking any situation and finding humor in it, and Rosalyn is simply one of the funniest women I've ever met. Our humor binds us together and makes our burden lighter.

Humor keeps all of us lighthearted. It's one of the reasons sitcoms like *I Love Lucy, The Cosby Show, Seinfeld,* and *Cheers* are so successful and popular—and why I routinely intersperse cartoons in my PowerPoint presentations during my lectures. Many times I don't read aloud what the cartoon says. I just stand quietly and smile as the laughter builds in the auditorium. Cartoons have an uncanny way of driving home the humor in our everyday lives and showing the lighter side of the human experience.

Although laughter appears to have the most significant benefit to your health, it's important not to overlook the more subtle but powerful effect of the smile. Smiling is a universal expression of happiness and friendliness, and we naturally gravitate toward people who are smiling and happy. We've been hardwired to do this because a smile means the other person is safe, and that the interaction with them will be nonviolent. But we now understand more about what's actually going on in the brain when we smile.

The part of the brain involved with reward and pleasure is called the nucleus accumbens, and brain surgeons have shown that when it's stimulated during surgery, the patient smiles and experiences feelings of euphoria. (Interestingly, many brain surgeries are conducted while the patient is awake, allowing the patient to communicate with the surgeon.) This response speaks to the convergence of motor and neural pathways and suggests that when we smile, we increase our sense of well-being. This happens, in part, because dopamine, the neurotransmitter of pleasure, is released—more proof that when we change our behavior, we can change our brain chemistry.

The bottom line is that humor is good medicine—good for our psyche, good for our health, and a good way to take life a little less seriously.

Relationships

⌒

No road is long with good company.
—TURKISH PROVERB

It was a busy day at my office in Las Cruces, New Mexico, in 1989. I was getting ready to go in for the third massage appointment of the day. I'd already talked to the client to determine what kind of treatment she was seeking and to gather some information about her overall health. She was in her early 20s, a student at New Mexico State University, and other than neck and upper back tension, she denied having any medical problems. I remember opening the door and hearing R. Carlos Nakai's haunting flute coming from the cassette player. The lights were dimmed, and the young woman was lying under a blue flannel sheet on the massage table. I worked the tense muscles in her neck, shoulders, and arms, and she began to relax. As I massaged her legs, I felt her shiver. I was covering her with a blanket, thinking she was cold, when I realized her body was shaking because she was crying. I put my hand on her arm and asked if she was OK. In words spoken so quietly I could hardly hear, she said, "I'm sorry."

I pulled up a stool, sat down, and spent the next five minutes listening to her story. She'd grown up in a small town in eastern New Mexico and had moved to Las Cruces the year before.

She'd gained weight since starting college, and a few months earlier she'd overheard the boy she liked joke to her classmates that she looked like a beached whale. They all laughed. She had no friends and felt isolated, sad, ugly, and very lonely. As her tears fell, I remember thinking that we lived in a town of 60,000 people and yet this beautiful soul had no one she felt safe confiding in but a massage therapist she'd never met before. As I finished the massage, I prayed my hands would convey the compassion and love in my heart. I hugged her as she left. She came in from time to time for a massage, though we both knew it was really for that human connection that feeds our soul and reminds us that we are not alone in the world.

I've encountered many lonely people over the years. I believe this loneliness of the spirit causes much of our suffering, and the treatment is not an herb or drug, it is relationship. Relationship, from the Latin *relationem,* means "bringing back" or "restoring." Being in relation restores our spirit, and brings us back to a community where we can feel safe and accepted. Without our clan, the loneliness and isolation can break our hearts, not just metaphorically but literally.

In 2004, the results of an international study—the Inter-Heart Trial, conducted in 52 countries with more than 27,000 participants—revealed that depression, social isolation, and a feeling of hopelessness increased a woman's risk of having a heart attack more than did diabetes, high blood pressure, smoking, or obesity. That's shocking when you think about it. As a physician, I was taught to measure blood pressure, monitor cholesterol, and counsel patients to exercise, maintain a healthy weight, and avoid smoking to reduce the risk of heart disease. There wasn't much emphasis on assessing the quality of a patient's relationships. But the science clearly shows that loneliness is as bad for our health as any of the more traditional risk factors. After reviewing 148 human studies on the effects of isolation on health, researchers at Brigham Young University found that being socially disconnected was equivalent to smoking 15 cigarettes a day or being an alcoholic. It is twice as harmful as being obese.

There are numerous reasons that persistent feelings of loneliness can be bad for our health. A lack of close interpersonal relationships impairs our immune system and adversely affects our nervous system, making it more difficult to handle stressful situations. According to John Cacioppo, director of the University of Chicago Center for Cognitive and Social Neuroscience, lonely people are more likely to use drugs and alcohol, exercise less, eat a diet high in fat, and have sleep problems, all of which are bad for health.

Prolonged loneliness turns on the genes that promote inflammation, which is a major driver of such chronic health issues as heart disease, stroke, diabetes, and cancer. Research published in prestigious journals, including the *Proceedings of the National Academy of Sciences* and *Lancet Oncology,* show that loneliness and psychosocial stress shorten telomeres, the protective coatings on the tips of our chromosomes, the structures that contain our DNA. As our cells divide over time, telomeres shorten and eventually cellular division stops. So, as our telomeres shorten, so, too, does our lifespan. Dr. Dean Ornish, a renowned cardiologist, has shown that comprehensive lifestyle interventions that include diet and meditation help prevent telomere shortening, and it appears maintaining close relationships can do the same.

Throughout history, our survival has depended on belonging to a group. The family and tribe provided protection against enemies, animals, and starvation, and care for the young, old, and sick. We all experience periods of feeling lonely at some point in our lives—that's part of being human—but loneliness is painful because we're hardwired for intimacy.

Using sophisticated brain imaging, Naomi Eisenberger, a professor at the University of California at Los Angeles (UCLA), found that when volunteers felt excluded by others from playing a game, the anterior cingulate cortex (ACC), the brain's alarm system, was strongly activated. The ACC is activated by physical pain, which is one of the most important indicators something's wrong. But the brain perceives psychological pain and social isolation exactly the same way.

What Eisenberger's research demonstrates, as do other studies, is that we literally *feel* the pain of loneliness. Because our survival has always been so dependent on our social attachments, the neural circuitry in our brain has been wired so that social isolation is experienced as real physical pain. Our alarm system is activated when we feel lonely, and we experience pain that is as real as any injury. In the case of loneliness, though, relief comes not from aspirin but from our connection to others.

Establishing healthy bonds isn't always easy for those who grew up in a family where they felt unloved, neglected, abandoned, or belittled. When this is what children learn, it makes it hard for them to trust and form lasting relationships. If this rings true for you, please consider seeing a counselor or therapist who can help you reframe those early experiences. But it can be difficult for anyone, even those who grew up in a loving home, to maintain important connections, because most of us are incredibly busy and relationships require time and attention.

Modern ecology and anthropology recognize that humans are part of a much larger web of life. This interdependent worldview is common in the cultures and philosophical constructs of many non-Western societies, particularly in Asia, Africa, South and Central America, and among indigenous North American tribes. These cultures place a very high value on the extended family as a source of resiliency and strength. Interdependent cultures see the needs of the individual as subservient to those of the group, and harmony is emphasized.

In many Western societies, though, the extended family is declining, as a result of high divorce rates and the increasing mobility of families. In independent cultures, like the United States, we're encouraged to be unique, competitive, and self-reliant. We learn to look out for ourselves and our immediate family members. But too much emphasis on the individual may come at the expense of meaningful relationships.

When my son, Mekoce, was in third grade, the difference between these worldviews was driven home personally. After scoring very high on several aptitude tests, Mekoce was placed in a "gifted" program, where he got A's and B's on his progress reports, along with "needs improvement" in class participation. About halfway through the school year, during a parent-teacher conference, his teacher expressed concern that Mekoce didn't raise his hand in class, even when he knew the answer. He didn't seem motivated to win in class competitions, even though she was confident he could do so if he tried. Although he was liked by his classmates and seemed happy in class, his teacher didn't think

Keeping Connected

- Time is one of our most precious commodities. Make your important relationships a priority. Don't take them for granted.
- Be thoughtful about who you choose to spend time with. Don't invest energy in people who make you feel bad about yourself or who you can't trust.
- Schedule something fun at least once a week. Invite friends or the extended family (grown kids, grandkids, or grandparents and cousins) to go on a picnic or hike. If getting together for dinner seems impossible, make a date for breakfast. Invite friends over for an afternoon of cards or board games.
- Keep the lines of communication open. Be a good listener. Ask others to tell you what's going on in their lives.
- Be aware of your stress level. Don't let all the anger and frustration build up over the day and then explode when your teenager talks back or your spouse forgets to pay the electric bill. Loved ones don't deserve your emotional garbage.
- If you need to widen your circle of friends, take up a hobby or join a class where you can meet people with similar interests. Volunteer at a local food bank, hospital, or animal shelter. Not only does serving others help us meet new people, it also can make us feel more grateful for our own lives.

"he'd get far in life if he didn't learn to be more aggressive and competitive."

I told her I believed learning cooperation and how to get along with others was more important than winning or showing you're the smartest kid in class, especially for young children. She looked me in the eye and said, "That's nice, but it's not the way the real world works."

I left feeling like a really bad mother. I'd always believed empathy, cooperation, and harmony were the keys to happiness and a good life. Maybe his teacher was right; maybe these qualities weren't compatible with success in the real world. After weeks of soul searching, I respectfully rejected his teacher's advice.

Years later, moments after winning the gold medal in tae kwon do at the Junior Olympics, Mekoce told his grandfather that even though he was happy to win, he felt bad for all those who didn't because they were just as good and had worked just as hard. My father wept. He told me he'd never felt more love or pride in his life.

I believe it is possible, and desirable, to see ourselves in relation to others as Mekoce did when he won. To truly "see" another allows us to experience and extend compassion and kindness. We feel connected, in relation to all of life, not separate or apart from it. None of the big problems we face today can be tackled alone. We can no longer afford to think only in terms of our individual needs. Whether we're talking about climate change, environmental issues, global economies, religious or racial intolerance, violence in our cities, the extinction of animals and plants, or the growing loneliness of human beings, the solutions can only come when we see ourselves as parts of the bigger whole.

Nothing and no one exists for long in isolation. As Chief Seattle, the famous 19th-century Squamish leader, said, "All things are connected like the blood that unites us all. Man did not weave the web of life; he is merely a strand in it. Whatever he does to the web, he does to himself." Among the Lakota people, the phrase *mitakuye oyasin*—"we all are related"—is still spoken repeatedly during prayers and songs as a reminder to reflect on our relationships with family, friends, colleagues, and those we've never met—and to think about our relationships with the animals and plants, for all life is connected and interrelated.

When you're feeling disconnected, go for a walk in the forest or along the beach. Light a candle and say a prayer for those who are sick or suffering. Look up at the stars or into the eyes of a child and take in the wonder of the universe. Experience awe. Strive to live in good relation and harmony with all creation. Don't spend your time praying to be thin or have more money—pray to be blessed with love, friendship, and contentment. For then, you will be rich beyond measure and feel alone in the world no more.

Words

Speech is the mirror of the soul; as a man speaks, so is he.
—Publilius Syrus

There's a story of a young girl whose best friend started spending all of her time with a new girl at school. Deeply hurt, the young girl decided to start sharing her old friend's deepest secrets with others and spreading rumors about her.

One windy autumn afternoon the young girl and her grandfather went down to the creek to go fishing. After putting their hooks in the water, the grandfather asked the girl to go put a hawk's feather at the top of the hill. She did and came back. A while later, he asked her to put an eagle feather by the big cottonwood tree down the creek. She did and came back. Time passed. No fish were caught. He asked her to put a turkey feather over by the road where the pickup truck was parked. She did and came back. She said, "Grandfather, why are we putting these feathers in all these places?" He just smiled, and they kept fishing.

Then he asked her to put a raven feather way over on a hill to the west. She did and came back. They ate the sandwiches that the grandmother had packed, and as dusk began to fall, the grandfather asked the girl to bring him all the feathers. She went to look for them, but the wind had scattered them about and she could only find one. The girl handed it to him and said she was sorry and that she should have put rocks on the feathers so they wouldn't fly away. He smiled as they packed up their stuff to go home. Standing on the porch, he took her hand and said, "Words are like feathers, child. Once you put them out in the world, they are blown about by the wind and very hard to get back. "

Like the young girl in the story, I have had times when I've not been mindful of my words. I remember snapping at my son once when he was five years old. It was the end of a very long day at the end of a very long week, and I'd picked Mekoce up from child care feeling absolutely exhausted. Mekoce was a bundle of stories anxiously waiting to be told. He chattered the whole way home in the car and then followed me into the bathroom, never coming up for air. Feeling totally irritated, I said crossly, "Mekoce, enough already! I have to go to the bathroom. Just go away and leave me alone for a minute!" He closed the door as he left.

After changing my clothes and freshening up, I saw him sitting on the floor in his room, back against the wall, crying. I knelt down to him. With tears streaming down his face, he said, "Mommy, please don't be mad. It's just that I wait all day to talk to you because you're my very best friend in the whole world."

I had lost my patience and broke that little boy's heart. I forgot that being in child care all day on sensory overload was hard on him, too, and how much he needed me to be present, truly present, at the end of a long day. That night we made a deal: He'd give me ten minutes all to myself when we got home each night, and after that we'd head to the kitchen

R
X

Wise Words

- ■ If you're struggling with a high level of negative self-talk, consider getting cognitive behavioral therapy. Go to *www.psychologytoday.com* to find a licensed therapist in your area.
- ■ Use positive affirmations to help reshape your thinking. The book *Affirmations: Your Passport to Happiness* by Anne Marie Evers is a great way to get started.
- ■ Watch the tone of your voice. Speaking gently will get far better results than shouting or using harsh words.
- ■ Be gentle with your criticism. As the cartoonist Frank A. Clark wrote, "Criticism, like rain, should be gentle enough to nourish a man's growth without destroying his roots."
- ■ The book *Nonviolent Communication: A Language of Life* by Marshall B. Rosenberg, Ph.D., will open your eyes to a new way of viewing language.

to make dinner together and talk. That way, we'd both be able to get what we needed.

That episode made it clear to me how easy it is to say things out of anger or things we don't mean when we're feeling stress—even, or maybe especially, to those we love the most. We cast those feathers out into the world, and we can never really gather them up again, no matter how often we say we're sorry.

Words are powerful. Words mean things. They allow us to communicate information, emotions, thoughts, and needs. Words can directly influence our health and well-being, especially the words we say to ourselves. Self-talk is that steady stream of thoughts that races through our heads everyday. "I'm happy, I enjoy my work, I have good friends"—these are all examples of positive self-talk. When positivism dominates our thoughts, we feel optimistic and hopeful. But negative self-talk—"I'm too fat, I'm stupid, I'm always late, no one likes me, I'll never have any friends"—can make us feel doubtful, pessimistic, anxious, or depressed.

The words we tell ourselves are often rooted in early experiences. If teachers or parents are highly critical, we may develop an exaggerated view of our weaknesses and have low self-esteem. If humiliation is used to teach or punish, we may believe we can't do things out of fear of failure or embarrassment. "Sticks and stones may break my bones but words can never hurt me" isn't true. Because of their power, words can belittle, hurt, and shame, and we may remember their pain years after they are spoken.

About a month after giving a talk at a nursing conference in Chicago, Illinois, I received my evaluation in the mail. The comments were very positive. Most said I was an excellent presenter and the information was relevant, which made me feel really good. Critiques such as needing to make my slides less wordy and use larger fonts were helpful and constructive. Then my eyes read, "What a joke. Someone should tell her it's hard to take anyone serious who looks like Cher. She'd be far more believable if she at least looked like a doctor."

There were roughly 300 comments on that evaluation from 1999, but that's the only one I remember. I went out and bought two black pantsuits and a pair of low-heeled black pumps to wear when I lectured. I pulled my hair back in a ponytail and wore a pair of small gold earrings. I was so nervous when I'd get up and present, worried about how I looked, whether I sounded professional. That lasted about six months until I finally realized I was trying to change who I was because of one anonymous comment on an evaluation! Why in the world did I put so much weight on those three sentences?

My Grandma Jessie used to say, "The devil's always looking for a crack." The devil is a metaphor for anything and anyone that finds your vulnerabilities or weaknesses and preys on them. My negative self-talk for a long time had included "high school dropout, divorced, single mom, failure." Reframing these negative thoughts was constant work. Yes, I'd dropped out of high school but later got my GED and went on to college and medical school. I was a divorced single mom, but that didn't mean I was a failure—just that I wanted more than an unfaithful partner. And being a single mom was hard but it wasn't shameful. Having my son was one of the greatest blessings of my life.

Yet the comment about my presentation preyed on my self-doubts at the time. I was inexperienced at speaking in front of crowds, and added to that were my early troubles with reading and speech. No wonder it didn't take much to rattle my confidence. The devil had found a crack.

It was hard walking up to the podium and speaking at the next conference. I was so afraid I'd forget my words, be embarrassed, and look ridiculous. Before I began my presentation, I would silently repeat three affirmations: "I am calm, I am confident, I am enough." But it took time to reframe the new negative self-talk, to tell myself that the criticism and judgment from that one comment on the evaluation belonged to the one who wrote it—it was never mine to carry in the first place. We have to be so careful not to let the negative messages of others become our own. For when we internalize them, we can find it harder to reach our full potential, take risks, and realize our dreams.

Words can create images, just like visual pictures. Many of us would find watching violent media all day very disconcerting. And yet, we are often unaware of the level of violent speech we are exposed to daily. On a societal level, we're barraged with aggressive speech. The deterioration of civil discourse is on bold display when listening to politicians and political pundits on both sides of the aisle. The rapid rise of violent lyrics in music is deeply disturbing. The news is filled with the war on terror, the war on drugs, the war on cancer, and the war on poverty. We're told to combat hunger, fight for the middle class and for peace, pick our battles, create a plan of attack, and shoot down our opponent's ideas.

As individuals, we can decide to embrace assertive over aggressive language. For instance, we could *work* to end hunger and poverty, instead of declaring war against them. We

℞ PRESCRIPTION FROM DR. LOW DOG

Words of Wisdom

A key virtue, according to Ben Franklin: "Silence. Speak not but what may benefit others or yourself; avoid trifling conversation."

can *cultivate* peace, instead of fighting for it. We can create a plan for *success,* and *offer alternatives* to our opponent's ideas, instead of attacking and shooting them down. We can choose to use words rich in praise and encouragement instead of ones full of judgment and criticism. Right now, we can opt to speak and listen with honesty, clarity, respect, and tolerance. We can pause before speaking and ask ourselves, "Does it need saying, is it true, and is it kind?"

Words are what move us through life. They mold and shape us. With deeper awareness, we can weave our words into a language of compassion that makes our own lives as well as those of our families and communities stronger, healthier, and more whole.

Forgiveness

Forgiving does not erase the bitter past. A healed memory is not a deleted memory. Instead, forgiving what we cannot forget creates a new way to remember. We change the memory of our past into a hope for our future.
—Lewis B. Smedes

Many years ago, two monks set out on a long journey. One day they came to a wide but shallow river. On the riverbank sat an old woman waiting to be carried across. She was shabbily dressed, her hair was matted, her teeth yellowed, and her skin gave off the foul aroma of one who hadn't bathed for many months. In an impatient tone she demanded, "Take me across the river! You fools—listen to me, I want to cross and I don't want to get wet!" The older monk walked into the river and crossed as if he had not seen or heard her. As the young monk started to follow, the woman yelled, "Carry me across the river, you idiot!" The young man turned around, picked her up, put her on his back, and carried her across. When he reached the other side, he gently set her down, and she walked off without a word or gesture of thanks.

The two monks continued on their journey in silence until it came time to stop and camp for the night. The older monk looked at the young man and said, "Why did you carry that foul woman across the river? You still carry her stench. It slowed us down and she offered you not a word of thanks."

R PRESCRIPTION FROM DR. LOW DOG
Cultivating Forgiveness

- Give yourself time. When you've been hurt deeply, it's important to allow time to work through the feelings of betrayal and anger. Don't bottle up your feelings. It takes time to heal.

- Give yourself space. It's sometimes necessary to distance yourself from the individual(s) who've hurt you, especially if there was any physical, sexual, or emotional abuse. Forgiving doesn't require reconciling.

- You don't have to forget. Some offenses are so great that it isn't possible to forget them. Accept that this might be the case for you. Over time, you'll find yourself blaming the person less often, and that takes away his or her power to continue hurting you.

- Trust and forgiveness are not the same. Although forgiveness is important for your health and well-being, it's not wise to trust someone who repeatedly hurts you. Move on. If you find yourself continually choosing relationships with untrustworthy people, get counseling, and find out why you're doing that.

- Forgive yourself. Sometimes, the person who is hardest to forgive is the one looking back in the mirror. Be tender with your own heart.

The younger monk sat looking into the fire and said quietly, "I picked her up and carried her across the river. Then I set her down. But you, brother, you have been carrying her for the past six hours."

They say that to forgive is divine, and it may be more important than you realize. Researchers are finding that forgiveness is beneficial for both our physical and mental health. At the heart of this research is the evidence that forgiveness reduces stress and all the adverse effects that go along with it. When we hold a grudge or harbor strong negative feelings toward another, our body reacts the same way it would to any major stressful event. Adrenaline and cortisol are released, elevating our blood pressure, heart rate, and blood sugar, all of which can spell trouble for our cardiovascular system and increase our risk for diabetes. Our muscles tense, and we experience more aches and pains. We get sick more often, as our immune response is suppressed. We feel more anxious and depressed. Blame, anger, and resentment—no one could really think these are good for our health in the long run.

Although this was unheard of 20 years ago, scientists today are actively conducting research to unravel what happens to the body when we forgive others. One thing they've found is that forgiveness is good for the heart. Charlotte vanOyen Witvliet, a psychologist at Hope College in Holland, Michigan, asked 35 female and 36 male students to relive lies, insults, and betrayals by friends, lovers, or family members, while they were hooked up to monitors that evaluated their stress response. Not surprising, their blood pressure and heart rate went up.

Think about the implications to your health if you frequently ruminate over painful experiences. Just as telling in this experiment, when participants were instructed to imagine forgiving the offenders, their heart rate and blood pressure dramatically fell. When researchers studied a group of people with coronary heart disease at the Veterans Affairs New York Harbor Healthcare System, they found that those with higher levels of forgiveness had significantly less anxiety, depression, and stress, and were less likely to suffer another heart attack when compared with those who were still holding on to the wrongs of their past.

But just like the monk in the story, it can be hard to let go of the hurt. Some of us carry the weight of the past our entire life. We hold on to the resentment even when we know it's hurting us and those we love. At first our anger feels justified. We may even feel like it gives our life energy and purpose. But we run the risk of getting trapped in blaming others for our circumstances, taking away our opportunity to focus on the life that we have. We get stuck. It can be hard to move past the pain, especially when the wounds are deep. Sometimes we don't want to forgive, because it feels like we're letting the other person off scot-free, or we confuse forgiveness with having to tolerate abuse or disrespect.

When my first husband was unfaithful, I was angry. I felt like he'd destroyed our family. I blamed him for making me a single mother. It took time to let it go, to surrender to the fact that I couldn't make someone love me or want to stay with me. It took time to forgive, even though forgiveness had always been readily extended within my childhood family. I had been taught and encouraged to forgive since the time I was a little girl. My Sunday school classes were steeped in messages of turning the other cheek and loving our enemies.

And for Christians, perhaps the most powerful example of forgiveness can be found in the moment of Jesus's deepest despair. Nailed to the cross and surrounded by those who cursed and wounded him, he said, "Father, forgive them; they know not what they do." I've always known that forgiveness is important and that it's not easy.

Over the years, I have spent many hours praying and meditating on forgiveness and compassion. Praying for compassion, which in Latin literally means "suffering," allows me to extend my love and care to others and to love and care for myself. I know that I am just a human being, complete with good and bad qualities. Seeing myself in this light allows me to hold others in the same light, and I forgive them for all the wrongs they have done to me, intentional and unintentional.

As I move through life, I've come to learn that forgiveness has more to do with our own attitude than with whether someone else is right or wrong. After my divorce, I knew that I didn't want to raise my son in a hostile, angry home or have him hear me say mean things about his father. I needed to move beyond my feelings of anger and blame so that I

PRESCRIPTION FROM DR. LOW DOG
Recommended Reading

For a book that helps you consider the advantages of forgiveness, read *Forgive for Good: A Proven Prescription for Health and Happiness* by Dr. Fred Luskin, director of the Stanford University Forgiveness Projects.

could continue on my journey. I had to take responsibility for my happiness. I didn't want to reap the fruit of bitterness. I wanted to plant seeds of compassion along my path and in the garden where my son played. And that's what I did, over time. Forgiveness is a process; it doesn't happen overnight.

If you're holding on to resentment or carrying the weight of your past, maybe you'll decide that now's the time to let it go. Is there someone you need to forgive? Sometimes it can be helpful simply to acknowledge the hurt. Tell someone that you trust what happened to you in that hurtful circumstance, how it made you feel, and explain why it wasn't OK. Giving voice to our hurt is often the first step to healing. Then choose to live in the present and to not relive the hurt you felt when you were five years old or the hurt from five minutes ago. If you repeatedly find yourself bringing up old hurts and telling the story over and over again, forgiveness is the only thing that will free you. The Aramaic word for forgive literally means "to untie." Forgiveness is what frees us from the ties that bind us to our pain and suffering. Forgiveness is what truly heals our heart and mends our broken wings so that our spirit can once again soar.

Animals

Until one has loved an animal, a part
of one's soul remains unawakened.
—ANATOLE FRANCE

When we talk about relationships, most of us focus on connections among people. Yet I feel it's incredibly important to understand the deep and powerful bond that exists between animals and humans. For many, pets are a part of the family. That has always been true for me. From my birth, I've been surrounded by animals—in all, I've had eleven dogs, three horses, and more than a dozen cats. My parents, particularly my father, loved animals and instilled in me a strong affection for them. It's in part thanks to my parents' attitude toward animals that I learned about loyalty, friendship, forgiveness, responsibility, and compassion.

Not only can animals help make us better people, but a large body of research indicates they can also be very good for our health. Studies show animals can lower blood pressure and stress hormones, ease anxiety, and increase socialization in both children and adults. But before I delve more deeply into the science, I'd like to share an experience that happened when I was a resident working in the emergency room at the University of New Mexico hospital.

A mother and child had been driving cross-country when the woman lost control of her car. The mother was thrown from the vehicle and died at the scene. The seven-year-old child, who had been wearing her seat belt, had only minor physical injuries. Because she had no family member with her and there were no beds available on the pediatric floor, we put her in a quiet corner in the back of the ER until we could get in touch with a social worker.

When the social worker arrived an hour or two later, the little girl wanted nothing to do with him or the stuffed animals he'd brought. She was scared, sad, and withdrawn. After a few minutes, a volunteer walked into her space with a big yellow dog wearing a bell around his neck. The girl, momentarily distracted from her fear, asked in a small voice, "Is he nice? Can I pet him?" When the volunteer said yes, she crawled down off the gurney and began to stroke the dog. When he licked her face, wagged his tail, and happily interacted with the little stranger, she smiled for the first time since she had come to the hospital.

Unlike any of us humans, this gentle creature was able to break through the girl's pain and comfort her. For a while, in the midst of her sadness, life was a little better and the world seemed a little less scary. I've never forgotten the little girl or the big yellow dog. It is a reminder of the powerful bond that exists between animals and humans.

I am delighted that we are seeing more and more specially trained animals being brought into hospitals, nursing homes, schools, and other settings. This is in part because of the growing field of animal-assisted therapy (AAT), which uses animals to improve physical, social, and mental well-being.

Research clearly shows that animals help us cope with lone-liness and chronic disease and make us feel less afraid. Some mental health professionals utilize AAT when helping trauma-tized children and adults talk about their experiences. Teach-ers and behavioral specialists have found that AAT increases positive social interactions and improves behavior in children with emotional or developmental disorders. And elders in care facilities with AAT or residential pets suffer less depression and anxiety. In general, studies show that 90 percent of hos-pitalized or institutionalized patients find AAT beneficial. And people who've had a heart attack and have a pet generally recover more quickly and live longer than those who don't. Animals can be so important to the severely ill that they have been described as "liaisons with hope"—whether they're cats and dogs or birds and fish. If you're interested in learning more about AAT, the Delta Society is a great resource.

Of course, for those of us who are not seriously ill, having a pet can still do great things for our health and add richness to our world. I believe that's due in no small part to the fact that pets give us unconditional affection and ask us to laugh at our overstructured, busy lives and come play with them. Even if I've had an awful day at work or school, when I walk in the front door, there's the dog wagging his tail and running up to greet me. No matter that I've been too preoccupied to take him on a walk for three days or have barely spoken to him while working on the computer. This forgiving friend looks up with eyes that say I am the most wonderful, special, amazing human being in the whole world. Or the cat greets me by rubbing against my legs, waiting for me to sit down so she can curl up, purring, in my lap.

R_X **PRESCRIPTION FROM DR. LOW DOG**
Experience Life With Animals

1. Adopt a Pet *(www.petfinder.com)*
    Petfinder is an online, searchable database of animals
    that need homes. It is also a directory of more than
    13,000 animal shelters and adoption organizations across
    the United States, Canada, and Mexico.

2. Train a Service Dog *(www.helpingpaws.org)*
    The mission of Helping Paws is to further the indepen-
    dence of individuals with physical disabilities through
    the use of service dogs. Volunteering with Helping Paws
    offers you a variety of rewarding opportunities. You'll be
    celebrating the human/animal bond while helping peo-
    ple achieve their independence.

3. Volunteer at an Animal Shelter *(www.humanesociety*
    .org/animal_community/resources/tips/reasons_volunteer
    _shelter.html) Make a difference in your community and
    help animals!

Caring for another living creature helps remind us that
we're not alone and eases the consequences of separation and
loneliness. But pets can also teach us about loss. I have loved
all of my animals and can tell you something special about
each one of them. But there was one that captured my heart
and never let go—our German shepherd Mato, named for
the Lakota word for bear. We took him to obedience school
and for long walks in the desert and mountains. I'd cook him

special dinners, and he'd take turns sleeping in our bedrooms. Mato was a big dog, pushing 130 pounds when full grown. He was loyal, intelligent, noble, and loving. He journeyed with our family through five household moves, home schooling, college, medical school, residency, and the birth of my daughter, Kiara.

One morning, shortly before his eleventh birthday, Mato tried to get up but couldn't. X-rays showed his right hip joint was essentially gone. He was given pain medication and we took him home, but it was soon obvious his time with us was coming to an end. Mato died as he had lived, surrounded by the people who had always loved and cared for him. We wrapped his body in a purple Pendleton blanket and buried it in the backyard of our home, near the cottonwood where he liked to sleep. But our friend and companion we buried deep within our hearts. I know that many of you have a similar story to share.

The animals we let into our lives help us grow in many special and beautiful ways. They not only teach us about unconditional love, happiness, joy, and companionship, but they also teach us about loss, grieving, and letting go. When their brief lives end and our hearts are breaking, we know we'll get through it because of all the wondrous times we've shared with them. We realize that ultimately the sadness was worth it. What an invaluable lesson—understanding that we can enter into a relationship we know will end one day and yet be unafraid. I believe that our lives, our health, and our human experiences are infinitely richer because of the unique relationship we share with the animals we love.

Play

We do not quit playing because we grow old;
we grow old because we quit playing.
—Oliver Wendell Holmes

Like most children growing up in the 1960s, I played every day. At school we couldn't wait until recess where we'd hang upside down on the monkey bars and play four square, hopscotch, tetherball, and jump rope. After school and during the summer, we'd chase each other in a game of tag, build elaborate forts out of old cardboard boxes, ride our bikes, go on treasure hunts, climb trees, and play kickball, hide-and-seek, marbles, and catch. There were no limits to our imagination; we could be anyone, anything, anywhere, anytime. We were pirates on a ship, damsels in distress, pioneers in a foreign land, teachers and firemen, cowboys and Indians, fairies and wizards. In the summer, we'd be at the pool from the time it opened until it closed, racing each other, doing handstands underwater, playing Marco Polo, seeing who could make the biggest splash off the diving board. We'd go outside in the rain and play in mud puddles or build snow forts and snowmen and have snowball fights. If it was too bad outside, we'd play games like Battleship, Risk, Clue, and cards.

Sometimes my mom would ask what I'd been doing all day and I'd say, "Nothing." With a puzzled look, she'd ask how

I could be doing nothing for the last four hours. I'd shrug and say, "I don't know." She'd just shake her head and go back to whatever she was doing. Maybe I didn't know how to describe it. Maybe I thought my mom had forgotten how to play. Many of us do forget, as we get older. We trade free play for 60-hour workweeks, family responsibilities, and countless demands on our time. We feel like there are never enough hours in the day, so we take the view that doing nothing is equivalent to being lazy.

PRESCRIPTION FROM DR. LOW DOG
Many Ways to Play

My favorite way to play is riding my horse, Kohana, alongside my husband on his horse, Ajax. We go for long rides in and around our property in the Santa Fe National Forest. However, we have many games that we play when company comes over or our children visit. Here's what's in Tieraona's game closet:

- Scrabble and Super Scrabble
- Balderdash
- Taboo
- Sorry
- Pick Up Sticks
- Boggle
- Rook
- Clue
- Three decks of playing cards
- Spill and Spell
- Scattergories
- Upwords
- Chess and checkers
- Monopoly
- Puzzles (too many to list)

Today, parents structure their child's entire life. From the time they rise until the time they go to bed, a child's every hour is filled with music lessons, school activities, soccer, homework, chores, and meals. Even play has to be planned. I remember when a mother asked to schedule a play date with my eight-year-old daughter. Play date? I didn't even know there was such a thing. When they arrived on Saturday afternoon, the mother asked what activities I'd planned for them. Planned? Activities? I said I was just going to let them play.

The woman left with a disappointed look on her face, and I went back to laundry and cleaning. The girls baked and ate cookies, ran around laughing outside, and painted each other's faces, pretending one was Belle from *Beauty and the Beast* and the other Jasmine from *Aladdin*. When the mother came to pick up her daughter and asked what she'd done all day, the little girl happily said, "Nothing." She was never allowed to come back.

The truth is that when children play, they're doing all kinds of things. Unstructured play teaches perseverance, problem solving, and social etiquette. We learn how to play together, share, and take turns. Play is the laboratory where we can experiment with being inventive, creative, and flexible. There's a lot going on, even though the time is not organized or heavily supervised. Although physical education and sports are important, they're not the same as play that has no purpose other than simply the joy of doing it. One of the things I loved most about playing when I was a kid was, with very few exceptions, the absence of parental involvement. No adults were needed to put together the game, make the rules, or supervise our every move. We'd play for hours, without any plan or destination in mind.

Maybe we become more risk-averse as we get older, afraid to make mistakes. Somewhere along the journey, we're taught that risks can lead to mistakes and that mistakes are bad. But without a certain amount of risk and mistakes, you can't learn, grow, or reach your full potential. Play encourages us to take some risks—and it teaches us how to assess them. It pushes us to the limits of our ability and causes us to mentally stretch and create new ways of doing things. We climb trees, fall out of them, and figure out a better way to get to the top. We go barreling down the hill on a bike, crash, and break a wrist. We learn about velocity and gravity without knowing any physics. The bumps, bruises, and mistakes are all part of life and learning. I fear that without play we may raise a generation

R_X PRESCRIPTION FROM DR. LOW DOG
Play 60

Being an NFL football fan, I want you to know that they have partnered with volunteermatch.com to help adults get involved in efforts to make the next generation of youth the most active and healthy.

Their website allows you to search for opportunities in your community that allow you to get active with sports and recreation organizations to help promote the message of getting active for at least 60 minutes every day. Visit *http://nflplay60 .volunteermatch.org.*

of people who have difficulty in dealing with the challenges of everyday life, have lost their creativity, and are so afraid to take chances that they never really experience the richness of life.

R̵X PRESCRIPTION FROM DR. LOW DOG

Play On!

Even though we're adults, play is still important, so make sure to build it into your life. Here's one secret—don't separate work and play:

- Play with your friends, families, and co-workers. It helps create trust and strengthens relationships. Put on some music and dance together in the living room. Go out bowling one night, head off to the park for a game of Frisbee, or enjoy a game of Putt-Putt golf. Don't make it about winning and losing, just play.

- Keep a deck of cards handy. You can learn to play dozens of games: crazy eights, rummy, spades, hearts, go fish! Our family loves to play Liverpool rummy and Rook, games we learned from our grandparents. The nice thing about cards is that you can take them anywhere and there are games for every age.

- Basketball anyone? You can put up a hoop just about anywhere. Going out to shoot a few hoops during a break at work is a great de-stressor. Playing H-O-R-S-E, twenty-one, or just practicing free throws is a great way to bond.

- Go for a swing. Playgrounds are great places to play with your children or to visit with a friend. Go swinging, hang on the monkey bars, or play on the teeter-totter. Laugh out loud.

- Have a charades night. Get together a group of friends and/or family and play charades. It's a great game to stimulate the imagination, and it can be played without keeping score.

- Do jigsaw puzzles. Pick a puzzle of a picture or landscape that you're drawn to. Then set up a dedicated puzzle table that can be left up for a while. The nice thing about puzzles is that you can work on them by yourself or with family and friends. It's hard to walk past the puzzle table without stopping for a while to see if you can find that one special piece. And if you love the puzzle, you can glue it onto a board, frame it, and put it up in the house.

Meditation

The more man meditates upon good thoughts,
the better will be his world and the world at large.
—CONFUCIUS

For the vast majority of us, from the moment we wake until the moment we fall asleep, our minds are racing. Positive and negative thoughts flit about, competing for our attention. Bodies tense and minds perplexed, we ruminate on the past and worry about the future. We can feel emotionally out of control, so overwhelmed by our lives that we become depressed. None of us would consciously choose to fill our days with anger, jealousy, or fear, but the reality is that many of us do. And when we fall victim to these emotions, it can make us say or do hurtful things to ourselves or to others, even to those we love.

In truth, there is a lot we can't control in our lives, and there are often no easy fixes for the problems we face. Disappointments, failures, heartbreak, sickness, and death will visit us all. Most of us were never given any tools to deal with the curveballs life throws at us. But the truth is, we *feel* angry or happy because we *think* we're angry or happy. Our thoughts drive our feelings. It's our perception that determines how we respond. Just as I believe the body is self-healing and health is its natural state, I believe the natural state of the mind is calm and clear. A well-trained mind is able to respond, not just react, to complex situations and problems. And meditation is one of the best ways to have a well-trained mind, to free our thoughts from all the chatter and noise that comes from the stress of our modern lives.

My first encounter with meditation took place in 1978, when I was studying the Korean martial art of tae kwon do. At the beginning of every class, we would kneel down, close our eyes, clear our minds from the busyness of our day, and focus only on our breath. For 3 to 5 minutes, we would center ourselves to prepare mentally for the 90 minutes of physically demanding exercise we were about to undertake. We finished class the same way. At first, I thought the whole thing was silly. I'd learned many things in my life without having to close my eyes and breathe!

Looking back, I know I resisted because it wasn't easy for me to quiet my very active mind. In fact, it was really hard. I struggled for months. I'd try to focus on my breath but find myself thinking about all kinds of things. I was training more than 20 hours a week, but instead of feeling relaxed, I was frustrated. Shortly after getting my red belt, I started pulling muscles and getting injured more often when sparring with my classmates. I was deeply worried about passing my black belt test later in the year, especially the part of the exam that required breaking boards with a flying sidekick. I felt like I was in a rut.

One day while eating lunch with Lorenzo Gibson, one of the black belts at the school, I asked if he would help me practice for the board-breaking part of the test. Having been one of my instructors for a long time, he said simply, "Tieraona, it's your mind you've got to focus. You have to expand what you think is possible. You have to let go of everything in that moment but you and the board." I took to heart what he said and realized that if I wanted be an accomplished martial artist, I was going to have to do more than train my body; I was going to have to discipline my mind.

I started reading any book I could find on meditation. I practiced focusing on a candle flame, which I found easier than focusing on my breath. After doing this a while, I found a local yoga teacher who was holding meditation classes in her home. I started going and learned to use the mantra *om mani padme hum,* a Tibetan prayer of compassion and blessings. Gradually, it became easier for me to stay in the present while meditating, and when my thoughts did wander, I simply observed them until they passed. My attention improved, and I felt happier, calmer.

PRESCRIPTION FROM DR. LOW DOG
Good Books on Meditation

- *Mindfulness in Plain English* by Bhante Henepola Gunaratana (free online at UrbanDharma.org)
- *Meditation for Beginners* by Jack Kornfield
- *When Things Fall Apart* by Pema Chödrön
- *Why Meditate: Working With Thoughts and Emotions* by Matthieu Ricard
- *Wherever You Go, There You Are* by Jon Kabat-Zinn
- *Change Your Mind* by Paramananda

When it came time for my first-degree black belt test, I felt physically and mentally prepared but also strangely unattached to the outcome. The forms and sparring went smoothly, and I barely remember running, jumping over three people, and breaking two inches of boards being held almost six feet in the air. The entire experience was transformational. The physical discipline of tae kwon do and the mental discipline of meditation changed forever the way I viewed the world around me—and the way I viewed myself. I could accomplish what seemed impossible if I was willing to put the full focus of my mind and body on the task and then surrender the outcome. It was an incredibly powerful gift for a 20-year-old woman.

The word *meditation* comes from the Latin *meditari,* which means "to engage in contemplation" or "to engage in reflection." Whether it has involved staring into the fire, listening to the sounds of waves, or moving to the hypnotic rhythm of a drum, meditation has always been a part of human life, spiritual practice, and religion. Kabbalah meditation comes from the Jewish tradition, the Sufi orders within Islam have a strong meditative focus, and the Holy Rosary and contemplative prayer are rooted in Christianity. The meditation most of us are familiar with in modern times is based in the formal Buddhist and Hindu practices of Asia and the Indian subcontinent. But although meditation was traditionally practiced for spiritual and cultural purposes, we don't need to adopt a belief in any religion or culture to practice it.

Today, increasing numbers of people are turning to meditation for health purposes. In the 2007 National Health Interview Survey, researchers reported that 20 million adults in the United States use meditation for stress reduction, relaxation, calmness, concentration, psychological balance, and general health and well-being, as well as to cope with illness and insomnia. The National Institutes of Health is investing millions of dollars into research on meditation, and the scientific evidence is showing that meditation can have far-reaching health benefits, in no small part because it reduces the deleterious effects of stress.

Researchers are also exploring the effects of meditation on the brain itself. We know through brain imaging techniques that regularly used neural circuits are strengthened and expanded, while those that are rarely engaged are weakened and contract. Think about it like this. If you use your arms to do heavy lifting every day, the muscles involved will get bigger and stronger. So if you decide you want stronger arms, you can start a training program using specific exercises that target specific muscles. Research shows you can do the same thing with your brain.

Neuroscientist Richard Davidson at the University of Wisconsin has shown that the brains of Buddhist monks who've logged more than 10,000 hours of meditation are fundamentally different from other brains. Using a brain scan called functional magnetic resonance imaging (fMRI), Davidson's team found that longtime meditators have greater activation of areas of the brain that are responsible for sustaining attention, processing empathy, integrating emotion and cognition, and perceiving the mental and emotional state of others. In other words, their brains have been permanently changed to be more attentive and empathetic.

Davidson's research, published in the *Proceedings of the National Academy of Sciences* and many other prestigious

Practicing Mindfulness

If you live in a town or city where there are meditation classes, you can ask to attend one to see if you feel comfortable with the teacher. Remember that meditation, like anything worthwhile, requires work and effort, repetition and discipline. That's why it's called meditation *practice*. If you've never meditated but would like to, the following pointers will help you get started:

- Start by sitting or lying down in a comfortable position in a quiet place where you will not be disturbed.
- Close your eyes and bring your full attention to whatever is going on around you. Notice any sounds. Notice if it is hot or cold.
- Bring your full attention to what is going on within you. Notice any thoughts or sensations in your body. Let them come and go.
- Become more and more still.
- Now bring your full attention to your breath. Breathe naturally.
- Notice how your chest and abdomen move when you breathe. Be aware of the air that moves in and out of your nose. Pay attention to the rhythm of your breath; notice if it changes but don't try to change or control it. Feel the rhythm of your breathing and gently settle into it.
- If you notice that your thoughts are moving away from your breath, gently bring them back. If you begin to feel

an emotion inside, gently turn back to your breath. Keep your heart soft.

■ Become more and more still.

■ If your mind wanders, if thoughts or emotions lead you away from your breath, gently return. Sometimes it will take longer to return to your breath, sometimes shorter. Don't judge the wandering. When you're aware that your thoughts are no longer on your breath, gently let them go, and return to your breath.

■ Become more and more still.

■ After 20 or 30 minutes, open your eyes and remain as you are for a minute before getting up. Notice how you feel. As you go through your day, take this calm state of awareness with you.

---

journals, has also shown that these same changes, though to a much smaller degree, occur in novice meditators after just an eight-week course in mindfulness meditation. When novice and experienced meditators were exposed to distracting noises during their meditation, those with the most experience had the least amount of neuronal response, indicating that it was much easier for them to remain focused. The implications of this research are enormous. One has to wonder how different our society might be if children were taught secular meditation throughout their years in school. Would they be less prone to violence? Would millions of children—and adults— no longer need stimulant drugs for attention deficit disorder?

The current scientific evidence is more than enough to convince me and many others in the field of medicine that meditation is a powerful tool for improving our quality of life in the 21st century. But I also believe in the benefits of meditation because I have seen it work experientially—in myself and in others. The 30 to 60 minutes invested in daily meditation pays enormous dividends: a sharper mind, clearer insights, and a greater sense of inner peace and connection with others.

Resiliency

~

*A man sooner or later discovers that he is the
master-gardener of his soul, the director of his life.*
—James Allen

Most of us spend at least 12 years going
to school, learning the three "R's": reading, writing, and arithmetic. Some of us
go on to college and maybe even gradu-
ate school, all so we can successfully enter adulthood and
the workplace. With all this education, more than 16,000
hours from first grade through high school graduation, you'd
think at least some of that time would be invested in teaching
us how to take care of our emotional and physical health.
Maybe it's time to add a fourth "R" to the classroom—resiliency. From the Latin *resili,* meaning "to spring back" or "to
rebound," resiliency is the ability to gather up one's strength
and resources to overcome adversity, and it's critically important for our health and well-being.

We are born with innate resiliency: Our DNA is programmed to adapt to a changing environment. This means
that all of us, not just a select few, are capable of overcoming
even severe adversity. Physicians often focus on the physical aspect of resiliency, while psychologists put more weight
on the emotional and mental components. As an integrative

physician, I believe that the health of our mind and body are inseparable. It's silly to think of the mind, or brain, as somehow separate from the rest of our body! It isn't. The brain, just like the body, benefits from optimal nutrition, regular physical activity, rest, and healthy relationships. When one or more of these are lacking, we are less able to withstand stressful situations. And stressful situations *will* come our way. Longfellow wrote, "Into each life some rain must fall, some days must be dark and dreary." My intention in writing this book is to show you how to optimize your life, so you can get through those dark, rainy days.

Because resiliency is a big subject, let's start with the role nutrition, exercise, and sleep play. Good nutrition is crucial if the mind and body are to functional optimally. The best way to ensure you're getting what you need is to eat a diet of minimally processed whole foods, as we talked about in the section on food. There's been a large body of scientific evidence showing that a diet of junk food is bad for the body, but now there's evidence that it's also bad for the brain. Researchers, who published their findings in the *British Journal of Psychiatry,* evaluated the diets of 3,500 office workers in England and found that eating a diet high in processed foods (sugar, fried food, refined grains) increased the risk of depression, while consuming a whole food diet (vegetables, fruit, fish) was protective. This isn't surprising when you think about it. Refined foods are devoid of many of the vitamins, minerals, and important phytochemicals (plant compounds) that contribute to the healthful benefits of richly colored fruits and vegetables, whole grains, nuts, seeds, and lean meat.

Processed, refined foods are also powerful promoters of inflammation in the body. Inflammation is necessary for our body to heal and repair itself, but in excess it increases the risk of blood clots, atherosclerosis, and insulin resistance. It has been linked to heart disease, diabetes, cancer, obesity, and now, it appears, even depression. People with depression have been shown to have high levels of C-reactive protein (CRP), a compound produced by the body in response to excessive inflammation. A growing number of researchers believe that inflammation may be driving depression, according to a report recently published in the journal *Medical Hypothesis*. So, not only is all the sugar-laden and refined food in our diet lacking in important nutrients, but it's also driving inflammation, which in turn is contributing to the enormous burden of chronic disease and possibly the dramatic rise in depression seen in many Western countries.

Another study in the *Journal of the American College of Nutrition* in 2011 found that, when compared with the general population, people with major depression and bipolar disorder are often deficient in folate, B_6, B_{12}, and zinc. Without folate, B_6, and B_{12}, our body can't make the neurotransmitters serotonin, dopamine, and norepinephrine, which are involved in mood or cognition. Many fruits and vegetables are good sources of folate and B_6, and fish and meat contain B_6 and B_{12}. Fish is also a rich source of brain-healthy omega-3 fatty acids, which lower inflammation. Fish oil and folic acid (folate) supplements have both been shown to improve depressive symptoms in human studies.

Zinc deficiency increases inflammation, reduces the responsiveness of our immune system, and may be linked to dementia, attention deficit/hyperactivity disorder and depression. Multiple studies show that zinc supplements decrease infections in children and adults. This is why, in addition to a healthy diet, I recommend taking a multivitamin and fish oil to fill in the "gaps." (For more in-depth information, please refer to the sections on food, vitamins and minerals, and omega-3 fatty acids in this book.)

There's no question that physical activity and exercise enhance resiliency. It's essential for our physical health, and a great way of relieving tension and stress and lifting our mood. I know in my own life, tae kwon do and tai chi were vital for getting me through some difficult periods. But more than being just a tension reliever, exercise can actually help us think better, allowing our brains to respond more efficiently under stressful situations.

It's been known for some time that exercise stimulates the creation of new brain cells, but researchers at Princeton University found that the brain cells formed during exercise are actually different from those created under sedentary conditions and are uniquely able to buffer the negative effects normally seen during stressful experiences. In other words, with regular exercise, you can make your brain more resilient at a *cellular* level over time!

And if you exercise outside, you might achieve even greater benefits. A review of ten studies with more than 1,000 participants found that green exercise—physical activity in nature— led to significant improvements in mood and self-esteem. The review, published in the journal *Environmental Science and Technology*, showed that the benefits are almost immediate; it only takes about five minutes outdoors to feel better. Again,

℞ PRESCRIPTION FROM DR. LOW DOG
Enhancing Resiliency

- Cultivate healthy, mature relationships. We all need people we can turn to for help and who can turn to us for the same.
- Spend time in nature. Take a couple of five-minute walks outside every day.
- Get organized. I have read and gifted to hopelessly disorganized friends both Sandra Felton's *Organizing for Life* and *Organizing From the Inside Out* by Julie Morgenstern.
- Make time for relaxation. Practice your breathing exercises every morning and night. Listen to soft, soothing music. Take a bath. Get a massage.
- Read something inspirational. *The Book of Awakening* by Mark Nepo and *Thirst* by Mary Oliver are two of my favorites.
- Get counseling if you're stuck. Cognitive behavioral therapy can help you reframe how you think about life.
- Make being active a part of your daily life. Join a yoga class, get a pedometer and work up to 10,000 steps a day, and stretch while you watch television.
- Write down one thing you're grateful for before bed: the grocery clerk who smiled at you, the spouse who made dinner or did the dishes, the child who loves you, or even the sun for shining. Practice gratitude.
- Eat healthy. Good nutrition will ensure your body is getting what it needs to function optimally. Take a multivitamin every day.

- Expect good things to happen. Visualize what it is you want in life.
- Be a lifelong learner. Go to a free lecture, join a book club, learn the names of all the trees in your area, or take a class that advances your career.
- Have faith that the universe is unfolding as it should. Accept that there are certain things you can't change. Find peace within the stillness of your own heart.

---

this isn't surprising. I know that going outside for five to ten minutes to "clear my head" always relaxes me. Just a short walk around the neighborhood or in a park can have beneficial effects on my state of mind.

Sleep and rest are also essential for resiliency. Researchers have been evaluating the effects of sleep disruption and insufficient sleep for decades, particularly when it comes to medical and aviation personnel. No one wants a pilot falling asleep in the cockpit or a doctor who hasn't slept for two days performing open-heart surgery. Research consistently shows that not getting sleep leads to more errors at work, increased risk of accidents, irritability, depression, reduced motivation, increased cravings for sugary and fatty foods, and higher blood levels of stress hormones and CRP. We all know that after a couple of nights of poor sleep, we simply aren't functioning at our best. I talk about this in more detail, as well as provide helpful tips, in the section on sleep in this book.

Now let's shift to a deeper exploration of what it means to be emotionally healthy. Our emotional health, or psychological well-being, is linked to our ability to handle stress, manage our emotions, have a positive view of ourself, maintain healthy relationships, and solve problems. Start with what many of us consider to be the primary cause of our woes: stress. Stress is neither good nor bad; it's how we *react* to stressful situations that determine their effect on our emotional and physical health. Imagine stress as a fire. When it's freezing outside, a controlled fire can keep us warm and save our life. But if that fire gets out of control, it can burn down our house and take our life. The fire itself isn't good or bad— it's how the fire is managed that matters.

We need a certain amount of physical and mental stress in our lives. Without the stress of gravity, our muscles would become flaccid and our bones weak. When the immune system is challenged, we develop antibodies that help us fight infections. But when the strain in our life overwhelms our body's ability to respond, we get sick and depressed. High blood pressure, heart disease, irritable bowel syndrome, headaches, insomnia, mood disorders, and even cancer all have at least some of their roots in the soil of excessive strain. It's not a job, friend, or bank account that's making us sick. It's not the stressor itself that's the problem; it's the way we respond to life's circumstances that counts.

There are thousands of stress-management books and classes in the marketplace. Many of them have to do with getting better organized. And it's true; chaos and clutter aren't good for resiliency, but there's more to it than that. Roger Epstein, a noted researcher and Harvard professor of psychology, has spent most of his career studying the impact of stress on health. In one large study, he found the people who are happiest and able to cope best are those who are pro-active at preventing stressful situations.

For instance, he found that those who planned their day or week to avoid or minimize stressors were far happier than those who used meditation or breathing exercises once they already felt overwhelmed with tasks and commitments. This is not to say that meditation and breathing aren't important parts of an overall approach to health and stress manage-ment, but proactively reducing stress is far more effective than reacting to it.

The second most important trait of resilient people in his studies was source management, the ability to schedule your time, organize your work environment, and delegate tasks. This means not taking on too many commitments and not always thinking that you're the only one who can do some-thing. "It's just easier if I do it" is a sure sign of someone who doesn't know how to teach and delegate effectively.

I've found these tools particularly effective in my own life. I do much better with a "to-do" list. By writing down every-thing that must get done, I am able to organize my days far more effectively, and it's incredibly satisfying when I'm able to check a task off the list.

Also, after years of feeling overwhelmed by the impossi-bly heavy workload I'd taken on, I started saying no—not easy for someone who wants to help, contribute, and please. But when I was honest with myself, I realized I didn't enjoy many of the things I was saying yes to. I started recommend-ing colleagues who could write and review articles, speak at medical conferences, or serve on committees. Although I was convinced the world would suddenly stop, lo and behold, committees still got their work done, conferences found presenters, and medical journals secured reviewers.

It was hard at first—my ego was bruised, because I wasn't nearly as indispensable as I'd secretly hoped. But as time went on, I found I had so much more to contribute. I realized saying yes to one thing inherently meant saying no to something else—no to hiking, cooking classes, reading a novel, or getting away for a weekend. When my life was tied up in all kinds of things I didn't really want to do, I had no time for the things I did want to do. As the stress lifted, my creative juices returned. My work improved and my presentations were more inspiring. When you feel like you're just keeping your head above water, all your energy is spent trying not to drown. But eventually, you become exhausted, and you have to make the conscious decision to sink or swim.

I use the analogy intentionally. As we look at an endless list of problems with no solutions in sight, we literally get a sinking feeling. If it feels like we have no control over a situation, it can be easy to lose hope. When there's no one we can turn to for help, we feel isolated and alone. The expression "sinking into depression" is highly descriptive. Our inability to cope positively with life's challenges puts us at high risk for depression and anxiety, which often coexist. In 2009, more than 40 million prescriptions were written for the anxiety drug Xanax, and in 2011, the Centers for Disease Control and Prevention reported that 11 percent of Americans over the age of 12 were taking antidepressant medications, a 400 percent increase from the 1980s.

In an attempt to stem this growing tide, researchers at the University of Pennsylvania have developed a program to determine if early intervention in elementary and middle school can reduce the risk of depression in adolescents. In 13 controlled trials, the Penn Resiliency Program was administered to more than 2,000 children ages 8 to 15, and the results showed that the program significantly prevents depression and anxiety, especially in kids with high levels of stress at baseline. The program consists of 18 to 24 60-minute lessons in which children are taught a variety of strategies for solving problems and coping with difficult situations and emotions. They learn how to be assertive without being aggressive and how to negotiate conflict and handle failure. They also learn strategies to promote relaxation. I love it—the fourth R! Hopefully, we can expand these kinds of programs so that our children learn reading, writing, arithmetic, and resiliency.

You were born with resiliency. No matter what you've been through, or are going through, within you is the ability to overcome adversity. You have the inner strength to get through those days when nothing seems to be going right or when all you can see are your failures and it's hard to remember your victories. There will be those dark nights of the soul, when our faith is tested and our confidence shaken. But through adversity, our character is shaped and formed. Avoiding or running away from challenges doesn't give meaning to our lives, but discovering our values and virtues as we struggle through them does.

This entire book is really about helping you find ways to enhance your resiliency. From the words you tell yourself and others, to the food you eat—your choices affect your health. You have the power to make different choices. Maybe you'll choose to meditate for ten minutes every morning or quit drinking sodas. What about choosing to take a five-minute walk outside during your lunch break or buying a book of inspirational quotes that you can keep handy? A journey of a thousand miles starts with a single step. Today, you can choose to make your life a priority.

Epilogue

CONTENTMENT

Be content with what you have; rejoice in the
way things are. When you realize there is
nothing lacking, the whole world belongs to you.
—LAO-TZU

WHEN I WAS 26 YEARS OLD, I spent a year preparing for a personal vision quest. As part of the preparation, I was to give away the possession that meant the most to me. I didn't have very much, living on about $4,000 a year, so at first it didn't seem that hard. I had my Ibanez guitar that I had dragged all around the country, playing with friends and even for supper one night at a restaurant in the Florida Keys.

As I sat strumming the worn strings that I knew so well, I realized that, although I loved my guitar, it wasn't my most important possession. After a week or two, I knew I'd have to give away my car.

It was a white 1963 Dodge Coronet that I'd bought for $400. It wasn't a great car, but it had four wheels and it got me wherever I needed to go. Who gives away their car? Surely, that was my most prized possession. But that night, I couldn't sleep. I knew deep in my heart that it wasn't my car that was so hard to give away. I knew what it was. I'd always known, but I didn't want to give away what I treasured. No one could expect me to give away something I loved so much.

For weeks I felt torn, until one day I walked into a friend's office and put my beautiful necklace in her hand, a richly colored turquoise pendant with two silver feathers coming off each side. I turned around in silence, walked out, got in my car, and wept.

A few days later I went to see my friend and teacher, Will Windbird. I told him I'd made a terrible mistake; the necklace was the only thing I had left from a family member whom I'd loved very deeply. From the day it was given, I hadn't taken it off. Now, I was living with my son and our dog in a little rental house with hardly any furniture. I had a beat-up old car, a guitar, and a few clothes in the closet. I didn't want to give up the one beautiful and special thing in my life. I wanted to get my necklace back and give away the car instead. Will listened gently, and as our conversation unfolded, I began to understand that the deep sense of loss and regret I was feeling wasn't about love or memories. I would carry those with me for the rest of my life. It was my attachment to the necklace itself that gave it so much power.

I learned a lot about myself during this process, not all of it pretty. If you'd asked me before the giveaway, I would've said I wasn't attached to my possessions. But in truth, even though I had little, I wanted what I had. I believed that my happiness was wrapped up in my stuff.

As I sat alone in the desert during my vision quest, it was as if the sun's intensity showed me that it wasn't my happiness that was wrapped up in my stuff; it was my suffering and my sadness. Happiness came from letting go.

On the second night of my quest, as I was looking up at the stars, it felt as if I were breathing the wind, and I felt my heart beating in the earth beneath me. When the sun rose on the third and final morning, I let go of the necklace and all it represented. And when I did, ever so softly, a sense of peace settled into my heart. As I walked out of the desert, I understood contentment for the first time in my life.

Contentment is being mentally and emotionally satisfied with the way things are. But how do you find it? How do you experience contentment? I think it starts by recognizing that our existence is marked with joy and sorrow, birth and death, health and sickness, times of abundance and times of scarcity, and then being willing to embrace it all fully. To embrace fully the richness of life, we must have a deep and abiding spiritual life, an unshakable knowing that we are part of something much greater than ourselves. When we feel separated from God, the divine, the Great Mystery, or whatever we envision that to be, we feel alone. As I've heard it said, Americans are physically overfed and spiritually undernourished.

When we feel alone and separate, we hunger and thirst for anything that will fill or numb the emptiness inside. Some turn to alcohol. I always thought it interesting that Carl Jung, the Swiss psychiatrist, thought that we called alcoholic beverages *spirits* because alcoholics had a greater thirst, or need, for the spirit. Some take drugs to ease the pain, and not just illegal drugs; one in ten Americans is on antidepressant medications. Do we really believe that all the sadness and depression we're seeing can be fixed by altering serotonin levels? Some of us eat to quench the craving.

The cake, doughnuts, and warm bread taste good, and we feel happy for a while. Then we find ourselves overweight and unhappy about the way we look. Some of us run up our credit cards, trying to buy our way to happiness, and then we feel ashamed because we're in debt and surrounded by stuff we really didn't want or need. Lying underneath all of this is our desire to feel inner peace and experience a more profound connection.

We experience contentment through a deep appreciation for the value and miracle of life. It's about letting go. It doesn't mean you can't work to improve your life or situation; it just means that you are capable of finding peace with wherever you are in your life.

When my Grandma Jo was 90, the doctor told her she would need to have a toe on her right foot amputated. It wasn't getting enough blood and had turned black. No one would be happy about having a toe amputated, but when I called and asked how she was doing, she laughed and said, "Honey, I'm doing just great. Anything less and I'd be cheating myself. How are you doing?"

My grandmother lived in the same little house with one bathroom and no garage for more than 60 years. She had a close circle of friends, young and old, and was active in her church. Like many people who live to such an old age, she had no real wants or desires. With her full mental faculties, and even as she was going to have her toe removed, she was content in her life.

Contentment is the beginning of real transformation. It springs from a place deep inside of us, from a sense of spiritual fullness. The paradox is that you can't pursue contentment.

There aren't ten easy steps to a contented life, though what is written in this book will help you create a soil where it can grow. Meditation, relationship, forgiveness, grace, nature, movement, love, and compassion will nourish the garden of your contentment, and one day, ever so softly, you will awaken to its glorious fruit.

Acknowledgments

This book was brought to life because of the generous sharing, mentoring, and encouragement that were freely given to me by friends, family, colleagues, and teachers. From the martial artists who helped me train my body and discipline my mind to the midwives, herbalists, and physicians who showed me the wonder and magic of birth, plants, and medicine—my life has been richly blessed. While there are too many to name, I would like to acknowledge a select few.

I want to honor all of the fellows, faculty, and staff at the Arizona Center for Integrative Medicine, particularly Victoria Maizes, M.D., Randy Horwitz, M.D., Patricia Lebensohn, M.D., Hilary McClafferty, M.D., Molly Burke, Moira Andre, Matt Stoner, and Rosalyn dePalo. A special thanks to April Gruzinsky, my friend and amazing assistant, who cheerfully keeps my life organized. I offer my deep and heartfelt affection and respect for Andrew Weil, M.D., whose vision gave birth to the field of integrative medicine and whose teachings inspire me. My love to those who dance with the plants and keep the noble tradition of herbal medicine alive: Rosemary Gladstar, David Winston, Roy Upton, David Hoffmann, Susun Weed, Aviva Romm, Tori Hudson, Mark Blumenthal, and the late Michael Moore. I offer my gratitude to Arthur Kaufman, M.D., and Alan Firestone, M.D., who taught me to be a compassionate and competent physician. With humility, I give thanks to Master Kun Jang Kim and Grand Master Myung

Kyu Kang for sharing the true meaning of what it means to be a martial artist. I am grateful to Karen Kostyal, who gently guided me through the process of taking my thoughts and experiences and putting them into written form, and to Susan Tyler Hitchcock and the entire team at National Geographic, without whom this book would never have made it to print.

And finally, I want to express my deepest love and gratitude for my family. For all those who came before and sacrificed much, so that I might have life. For my beloved husband, Jim, and my beautiful children, Mekoce and Kiara. I fall in love with each of you over and over again. You are my inspiration, my sunshine on dark days, my most delightful companions, and my very reason for being.